The Power Within

FROM NEUROSCIENCE TO TRANSFORMATION

Alane Daugherty, Ph.D.

California State Polytechnic University, Pomona

KENDALL/HUNT PUBLISHING COMPANY
4050 Westmark Drive Dubuque, Iowa 52002

Printed in the United States of America
10 9 8 7 6 5 4 3 2

DEDICATION

For Michael and Sammy

ACKNOWLEDGMENTS

My work and my passion are one, but my work could not, and would not exist without the foundation upon which it is built. I am deeply grateful for the work of those whom have inspired me and encouraged me to take this path. Many of the authors cited in this text, just by the nature their work, have changed my life forever. Thank you.

Thank you, also, to Molly Soto. Your many hours of assistance, hard work and cheerful disposition helped me turn a seemingly insurmountable task into a proud accomplishment. I am very appreciative.

Finally, I extend sincere appreciation to David Drew. When I look up the definition of appreciation I find "a feeling or expression of gratitude." When I look up the word gratitude I see "a feeling of being thankful to somebody for doing something." Your support and encouragement came in so many different forms throughout this process I feel the terms gratitude and appreciation should have exponents attached to them. Thank you. . . .

CONTENTS

PART ONE
PHYSIOLOGICAL FOUNDATIONS OF NEGATIVE AND POSITIVE INTERNAL EXPERIENCE

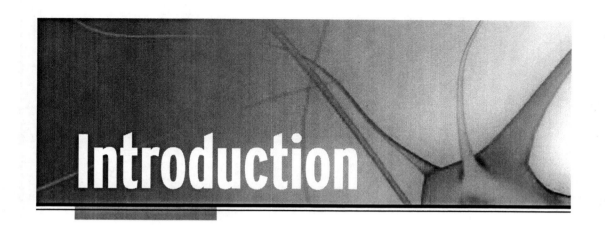

Introduction

The Importance
of Internal Experience

CHAPTER one

Looking Inward

Introduction

"You have been facing the wrong way!"[1] I read those words in a book on discovering the sacred in ourselves, and reading those words changed my life. Not only did those seven words give me the literary description of what I intuitively knew to be true, they launched an academic and personal journey that has become my life's work.

This book is about transforming the stress and chaos in our lives by looking inward. It is about understanding the detrimental physiological and biochemical effects of stress and anxiety on our bodies, minds, and souls, and, conversely, the significant and beneficial effects of love, gratitude, and appreciation. It is about the fundamental importance of internal experience and understanding that we have a choice of how to live our lives and a wealth of resources waiting inside each and every one of us to help us do so.

This book is about what I have learned academically and personally. It is rich with what I have learned through a passionate exploration of the subject matter as a doctoral researcher and through my relationship and experience with many university students and other students of life. This book is about understanding the science and the choice of transformation, neither of which will happen without a willingness of experience. This book is about the miracle, scientific and personal, of looking inward.

Background and Rationale

As a doctoral researcher I was taught to be candid and straightforward about any biases I may bring into my work, and I would be remiss at this point if I did not, in all honesty, share the following convictions.

I perceive myself to be fundamentally a spiritual being; I trust my intuition. I believe that deep within each of us lies an entirely awesome source of inner radiance, a reliable source of wisdom to help guide our lives. It is imperative that we learn how to listen. I believe most of us live our lives looking "without" for answers and constant validation of whom we think we should be, waiting for the world to provide the anchor we cannot provide for ourselves. This need for validation becomes insatiable because we always feel there is something missing, something more we need to be.

This reliance on our "external life" has left most of us feeling empty, chaotic, unanchored, and searching for that "next fix," because we believe the next fix is the one that will assuredly bring us happiness. I believe that the evolution of our culture to be primarily externally based has resulted in a society out of touch with and without reverence for the cultivation of the internal self. Gandhi said, "What is Truth? A difficult question, but I have solved it for myself by saying it is what the voice within tells you." That voice within me tells me that the cultivation of the internal self is of paramount importance if we are to live lives as whole human beings.

Externally based living pervades academia. The internal, or spiritual, dimension of our lives has traditionally been regarded as intensely personal. The innermost component of who we are has been deemed an inappropriate exploration in academia.[2] Yet, in a 1998 Gallup poll, 82 percent of Americans expressed a need to experience spiritual growth.[3] Given this state of current academic thinking, is it possible to suggest a fundamental shift to include internally based living within the academy?

My friend Alexander Astin, from the Higher Education Research Institute (HERI) at UCLA, argues that Liberal education was originally grounded in the maxim "know thyself," and yet the development of our internal selves receives little attention in our universities. Furthermore, he argues, a cursory look at our higher educational system makes it clear that the time devoted to the exterior as opposed to interior aspects of our lives has gotten way out of balance, a balance we need to correct.[4]

I deeply believe in the previous philosophical discussion and the tenants of Dr. Astin, and I would argue that in no other discipline has the external vs. internal gotten as out of balance as it has in health and wellness. I believe there should be no question regarding the appropriateness of the cultivation of our internal lives in the areas of health and wellness. Transformation of stress and anxiety, and the transformation of self cannot even begin without a look inward. Fascinating advances in neuroscience and positive psychology are validating this point with overwhelming evidence. Our bodies, minds, and souls transform when we feel positive loving emotions. Our internal experience, through a complex process of physiological adaptations, eventually becomes who we are, and the external experience we live.

While my personal tendencies and biases have certainly guided the direction of my pursuits, I am equally passionate about having my work based on scientific and experiential truths. I believe knowledge is power. Understanding from a scientific standpoint how our bodies respond to stress and anxiety and, conversely, positive loving emotions gives the foundation necessary to inspire change. According to Lama Surya Das, Tibetan Buddhists believe that at the heart of you, me, and every single person is an inner radiance that reflects our essential nature, which is always, utterly positive.[5]

New science and neuroscience are beginning to show us that getting in touch with this innermost aspect of ourselves and acutely feeling its presence in our lives creates measurable biochemical, neuroscientific, and even anatomical changes that determine who we are and how we function in the world. This book was inspired by my passions, yet it is based on scientific exploration. This exploration includes the examination of acute stress and anxiety, a scientific exploration of cultivating positive emotion, an experiential, critical look at what holds most people back from true transformation, and suggestions for overcoming those obstacles. In short, it looks at the power of internal experience on the quality of our lives, it examines how destructive negative internal experience can be, and it explores the vast possibilities of intentionally cultivating positive internal experience.

Overview

This book is built on several premises:

- Most of us live our lives out of balance, consumed with stress, anxiety, and chaos. We feel out of control without an internal anchor.

- Our constant exposure to this stress and anxiety perpetuates itself and causes very real biochemical, physiological, and damaging brain reaction patterns that literally become who we are and how we perceive our world.

- At the heart of every human is an inner radiance, a source of internal strength and wisdom. Connecting with this positive internal experience is usually felt as a positive emotional reaction, internal coherence, or deep resonance.

- Because of the chaotic nature of our lives, most of us live in such a way that we can't connect with this type of positive experience or even realize its potential presence in our lives. On a biochemical and neuroscientific level, these states are in direct opposition to each other. How can you follow your heart if you can't even hear it?

- Intentionally cultivating internal experience based on higher emotions produces profound and fundamental changes in our physiology, biochemistry, and brain reaction patterns that change our whole way of being in the world.

- Even though most people profess to want change, most sabotage their own efforts because they are familiar with the chaos and are not truly willing or ready for deep change.

- Transformation can only occur when we examine our willingness, at a deep level, and take concrete and experiential steps toward change.

Transformation

The underlying theme of this book is that the answer to transformation of stress and anxiety must come from within. In our internal selves we have an inexhaustible source of wealth and power. Dr. Wayne Dyer defines and breaks down the term *transformation* (trans-form-ation) as "using action to move beyond our current form."[6] I sincerely believe that to truly motivate people to change they must first have an understanding of how destructive their current thought patterns and "habits of feeling" are to their personal growth and day-to-day existence.

We tend to think life is just something that happens to us, and we spend most of our time being reactive instead of proactive. If we are accustomed to the concept of proaction, it is typically externally motivated, prompted by the illusion that we can somehow force our life into attunement by the external actions we take, regardless of our emotions or the state of our feelings. If we understand from a scientific standpoint the damaging and harmful effects of allowing ourselves to wallow in negative emotional states and the beneficial and constructive effects of cultivating positive emotional states through our thoughts, feelings, and relationships, we can begin the process of moving beyond our current form.

The Power of Emotion

Positive or negative, emotion has power. Appropriate emotion is a healthy thing, but all too often we choose to stay in negative emotional states that no longer serve us. We constantly keep our attention on all the things that go wrong or could go wrong; we keep grudges and speak through damaging and hurtful language; we choose to hate or act out of envy; we put ourselves down and allow ourselves to be victimized by our past or present.

Every time we have an emotional reaction, we produce a cascade of biochemical effects that literally affect our whole body. In addition to the biochemical effects, we cultivate and strengthen brain reaction patterns to match that emotional state. The longer and more often we expose ourselves to those reaction patterns, the stronger they become. In addition to strengthening brain reaction patterns, our current emotional and mood states tend to stimulate similar subconscious brain reaction patterns, intensifying and perpetuating our current emotional state. We literally train ourselves to experience more of the same.

The positive aspect of all these physiological reaction patterns is that they also respond to positive and loving emotional states. If, as Lama Surya Das purports, every single person has an utterly positive inner radiance that reflects our essential nature, keeping our emotional attention on this radiance should have profound implications for the way we live. When we reflect this radiance through our thoughts, feelings, words, and relationships, our internal experience changes, and our bodies, our psyches, and our lives adapt to what we give to them and cultivate more of the same.

Internal Attention and Internal Experience

It is my opinion that most stress and anxiety comes from living in an internally chaotic place and being out of sync with what we know to be internally or intuitively true. Stress itself is like the static of an out-of-tune radio receiver: All at one time the static prevents us from clear internal hearing; conversely, clear internal hearing prevents us from the distractions of the static. The "Catch 22" in this scenario is that if our lives are full of the static of stress and anxiety, it is a challenge to tune into this internal part of ourselves, and yet tuning into this internal part of ourselves may clear the static of stress and anxiety.

Thus is the cyclic nature of the psychophysiology of emotion. Feeling internally chaotic and cut off, from a biochemical and physiological level, produces more of the same. Conversely, feeling internally coherent and emotionally grounded also produces more of the same. The answer to this seemingly contradictory state of being may be in awareness. There is power in the awareness of the detrimental effects of stress and anxiety. There is more power in the awareness that cultivating higher emotion through intention, practice, and true willingness may break this pattern and change our lives. The key may lie within.

Lack of internal attention creates chaos. Dr. Jennifer Lindholm, also from HERI, found that 75 percent of incoming college freshmen across the nation feel a lack of internal development. This statistic was garnered through a comprehensive questionnaire administered to 112,000 entering freshmen at a nationally representative sample of colleges and universities. Additionally, even though three-fourths of students reported feeling a greater need for internal development, 62 percent reported their professors never addressed such issues.[7]

Given the magnitude of these statistics, it is not surprising that the American College Health Association (ACHA) has identified student stress as its number one detrimental health issue and combating student stress as its number one goal. Yet, we are still looking externally for answers.

The Importance of 'Feeling' Attention

A major premise of this book is that where we keep our "feeling" attention is a major determinant of our emotional state, and our emotional state is the major determinant of the stress and anxiety we experience on a day-to-day level. Major advances in our understanding of the neuroscience of the emotional brain support this premise. As will be discussed extensively throughout this book, the neuroscience, biochemistry, and electricity of emotion greatly influence the rational mind and, according to R. Joseph, men and women remain creatures of emotion.[8] Moreover, in his book *Synaptic Self,* Joseph LeDoux, a leading researcher in brain synapse patterns and emotions, argues that the brain synapse patterns created and strengthened by repeated emotion literally become who we are.[9]

If man and woman remain creatures of emotion, is our emotional state, and thus our anxiety level, predetermined? Three major findings in the field of neuroscience in the past several years offer a resounding "no." The adult brain was previously believed to be rigid;

that is, once the neural synapses were developed, they became permanent and basically determined who we were. In addition to believing that patterns of brain activity were set, scientists believed that there were individual differences along the eudaemonic scale, a baseline spectrum of happiness; where we fell on that scale was essentially determined by our preset brain activity.

However, new medical technology and our ability to literally see changes in brain functioning have shown that the human brain possesses what we call *neuroplasticity*. Neuroplasticity is the ability of the human brain to change its structure and function in response to the specific firing patterns to which it is routinely exposed. In other words, every time we have an emotional reaction or choose to keep our "feelings" fixed in a specific state, our brain firing patterns strengthen for creating more of that state. As will be shared in more detail later in this book, the process of emotion may start as a feeling state. Antonio Damasio argues in *The Feeling of What Happens: Body and Emotion in the Making of Consciousness* that our feelings create our emotional reactions.[10]

The second major finding in neuroscience showing that our stress and anxiety levels are not preset is that certain forms of mental training, specifically invoking positive feeling states, have been shown to change both neuronal activation and neuronal circuitry.[11] In other words, through certain types of mental training not only can we teach our brain to fire differently, we can bring about foundational changes in its circuitry. According to LeDoux, these circuitry patterns ultimately determine who we become.

A third finding comes from Dr. Bruce Lipton, a former medical school professor and research scientist who questions our previous understanding of genetic predetermination and DNA. In *The Biology of Belief,* Lipton argues that genes and DNA alone do not control our biology. Instead, he contends, specific genetic patterns and DNA are activated, or not activated, by biochemical and energy signals outside the cell. These chemical and energy signals are received by the cell's receptor sites and thus alter its function by their influence on the genetic codes within the cell. Most importantly, these chemical and energy signals are a response to our positive or negative thoughts or feelings.[12]

Given what we now know about the neuroplasticity of the brain, the relationship between stress and anxiety and where we choose to keep our feeling or emotional attention should be apparent. The internal experience of these states creates the cascade of reactions and adaptations throughout our bodies and brains. One point needs to be completely clear at this juncture: Appropriate emotion is healthy and should not be suppressed. However, choosing to keep our attention in a negative feeling state, to ruminate or catastrophize long past any positive expression, is detrimental to our emotional and physical health. Ultimately, those choices become the way we operate in the world. Moreover, gaining an understanding of emotion and brain reaction patterns helps us more clearly define and grasp what is an appropriate emotional response, as opposed to a conditioned emotional reaction.

Chaos vs. Coherence

If where we keep our feeling attention translates to our emotional state and the state of our internal experience, and if the statistic that 75 percent of college students feel a lack of internal development is correct, it is not surprising that most of us live from an internally chaotic place. From that place, we can't help but experience stress and anxiety on a daily basis, with all the resultant negative brain adaptations. What is an internal life? What does the development of an internal life have to do with reducing stress and anxiety and developing emotional resilience? The two terms that come to mind in response to these questions are internal coherence and internal integration.

Most people, when asked how they experience stress, ultimately describe a feeling of emotional or internal unease. This unease may be in response to a specific trigger or experienced as a general feeling. Most of us live our lives thinking the answers are external; we are always searching for something more when our internal lives remain in chaos. We think that the internal unease we are feeling will be diminished when we achieve something more, buy something more, do something more.

If we now know that the neuroscience of emotion basically determines our level of happiness, we are beginning in the wrong place by searching for happiness externally. Outside circumstances may affect our emotional state, but unless we first pay attention to our internal emotional state, those circumstances probably won't appear, or we won't recognize them when they do. Furthermore, if those circumstances do appear and we remain in an emotionally chaotic place, complete with the accompanying detrimental brain patterns, we will begin to sabotage those circumstances.

How do we begin to look inward? I personally love the description of how Michelangelo came to sculpt the statue of David. He said that as he chipped away at the marble, he removed all of the pieces that weren't David, and David began to appear. The presumption of this book is that if we can cut through enough static, stress, anxiety, and chaos by turning inward, what lies at our internal core is a perfectly loving and compassionate state. If we can begin to focus our attention on and routinely experience this internal state, our brains change, our biochemistry changes, and the way we function in the world changes.

Admittedly, as will be discussed in depth later in this book, many of us have painful, angry, and anxiety-laden emotional reaction patterns buried deep within our brains. These feeling state reaction patterns are activated subconsciously, which makes looking inward a scary process. Instead of finding a perfectly loving and compassionate state, we find fear, hurt, and anger. I deeply and sincerely believe that understanding how these reaction patterns are activated is the first step in diminishing those patterns, as knowledge and awareness begins to diffuse the fear and negative reaction. Furthermore, once those negative reaction patterns begin to be diminished and replaced by positive reaction patterns, it is easier to connect with the love behind the fear.

The Semantics of the Internal Self and Internal Experience

What is an internal self? What specifically comprises internal experience? The academy, unless specifically related to theology or philosophy, goes out of its way to avoid terms like *soul, spirituality,* and *internal self,* and people seem to have many different comfort levels with using these terms. In his book *Care of the Soul,* Thomas Moore says "shrinking the soul to manageable size" is our era's preoccupation.[13] Whatever words we use to describe its essence, there seems to be a reluctance, even a fear, in academia to acknowledge its presence.

However, in addition to the data on college students, a 1998 Gallup poll revealed that 82 percent of Americans expressed a need to experience spiritual growth. This statistic had increased from 54 percent only four years earlier.[14] If that trend continues, that statistic may be even higher now, and neuroscience is showing that the experience of spirituality is measurable in the brain. Avoiding terms like *soul, spirituality, internal experience,* or *internal self* and shunning the exploration of this subject matter may be denying a necessary and desired component to our psychological, emotional, and physical health.

Still, semantics—that is, the words we use to describe something—are powerful, and the semantics of internal experience can be especially problematic. Some will equate internal experience with spirituality, others will not. When the terms *spirituality* or *soul* are used, they are quite often confused with religious dogma, which is a very different concept and may have many negative connotations associated with it. Thus, the terms *internal self* and *internal experience* are used intentionally in this book to emphasize a universal aspect.

Some define for themselves the internal self to be a source of connecting with a deity, a universal source of love or a specific religious figure. Some choose to define the internal self as the deepest parts of themselves. Many fall in between. The semantics and definitions aren't important. In fact, I believe our interpretation of the internal self is somewhat ineffable.

I have become quite fond of the term *ineffable.* I first discovered this word in *Ask and It Is Given* by Esther and Jerry Hicks.[15] *Ineffable* basically means that something cannot be described in words; the minute we try to ascribe words to define it, we begin to lose the essence. It is almost an intangible state of feeling. We may not know how to describe it completely, but we know it because we can experience it.

The deepest parts of our internal selves are ineffable, and we should use whatever terms we feel comfortable with in this context. The absolute key in the description of the term *ineffable* is that we know it because we feel it. It is a feeling state of being. If somehow we can teach ourselves to tune into our internal selves, this ineffable essence that lies at our core, our emotions change, our brains change, our biochemistry changes, our relationships change, and our world changes. Our internal experience eventually becomes who we are. Again, because of the cyclical nature of emotion, small steps to transformation can begin to reverse the process of stress and anxiety and replace those patterns with calm, centeredness, and connection.

The Power of Psychophysiology

I choose to use a scientific and physiological basis to describe what happens when we turn inward and intentionally cultivate a higher emotional feeling state and, conversely, what happens when we live from a chaotic anxiety-laden state because I believe scientific understanding helps to motivate. When we understand that the emotional unease we are experiencing has a physiological basis and perpetuates more of the same, we can better see the extreme harm we are causing in our lives when we choose to remain in those states too long. We can understand from a scientific standpoint why it is better to love than to hate, why it is better to focus on abundance rather than lack, why it is better to connect than reject. We can understand that we have the power to transform the stress and anxiety in our lives and live more productively and happily.

Although a major part of this book relies on the neuroscience behind stress and anxiety and, conversely, positive emotion, the mind, soul, and body cannot be separated. Quite often we hear people say things like "Listen to your heart," "What does your gut say?" and "I need to sit on it." Examining our reaction to these statements most often manifests itself in a feeling state of knowing.

Another topic we will explore in this book is the physiological impact of emotions. In her extensive work on the "molecules of emotion," Candace Pert says neuropeptides of emotion are released throughout the body, and every cell has receptor sites for those peptides.[16] The Institute of HeartMath has showed the electrical impulses of the heart reflect a very different sine-wave pattern when we experience appreciation or frustration.[17] Tuning into our internal self affects every part of our physical, psychological, and spiritual being.

A large part of this book is on the science of stress and anxiety, and, alternatively, the science of developing emotional resilience. The scientific foundations explored in this text are from a large body of literature, from which I have tried to present important points in an understandable and pertinent manner. I wish I could say discovered the science myself, but I did not. The information and answers are in the scientific literature; however, I have synthesized several sources to substantiate my claim that stress and anxiety can be replaced by positive, loving, and higher emotions and that in doing so we can change our lives substantially.

Although the scientific validation of these truths may be new to some, the message may not be.

The Question of Willingness

It is my experience that in numerous areas of personal change or self-transformation, the answers to many problems are available, yet they are not utilized. My fundamental belief is that what prevents most people from substantial change is a true willingness to live differently. Although the willingness to do what it takes to achieve a goal, in an external sense, may also be an issue, I believe it also takes willingness to receive.

Most of us live lives so fraught with stress and anxiety that those states of being become a familiar place—not a healthy or comfortable place, but familiar. We are, on a psychological and physical level, addicted to stress. We think we want to live differently, but at a very deep level we are not really willing to do so. The status quo has become comfortable. It has become what we are.

My friend Violet Scolinos grew up in the United States, moved to Europe, and lived for a while on an island in Greece. After she returned to the United States, we talked about the differences in the cultures. Though she is familiar with the American way of life, she was having a hard time readjusting to its pace. She said it feels as if everyone is addicted to a life of running on a frantic treadmill; they are afraid to get off the treadmill because if they do, they will have to actually look inside themselves.

The foundation of this book is built on the concept that looking inward is the only place we will find peace and calm the emotional unease to which we are so accustomed. It is also about the very real physiological and biochemical changes that take place when we intentionally and regularly make an emotional shift to a positive and loving state and the higher potential we can achieve when we do so. The question of willingness, however, looms large. It is my experience that a large number of people resist looking inside because they are afraid what they will discover. Ironically, it is this reluctance to look that causes most of the stress and anxiety.

When most people hear the term *stress management,* they have this concept that the discipline is about organizing themselves to such an extent that they can be more functional in the external world without ever looking inward. Their goal is to continue to live this chaotic life but feel better about it. Steven Covey uses the metaphor of spending all your time and energy climbing "the ladder," but when you get to the top, you realize it is the wrong wall. He argues that the most successful people are willing to go inward first to make sure the ladder is where it is supposed to be, according to who they are at the deepest level. Then climbing the ladder is easy.[18] It is my belief that the ladder will appear if you are waiting at the right wall and if you are genuinely ready and willing to accept it.

Dean Ornish also has a metaphor that is fitting for this concept. He likens coronary bypass surgery to the way we live our lives every day. He suggests that we have literally and metaphorically blocked the channels to our heart by our own behavior, and we play out this scenario every day in heart surgery. Instead of focusing on developing ways to keep our heart channels clear, we perform numerous bypass surgeries, made necessary because we have lost the important connections to our heart.[19]

Our Journey as a Labyrinth

The arrangement of this book is very much like a labyrinth. The labyrinth is an ancient symbol built on the image of a spiral as a meandering but purposeful path in which one walks. The labyrinth is a metaphor for the journey to our own center and out again into the world.

Because the path is circuitous, many people confuse labyrinths and mazes, but there are fundamental differences. The maze has twists, turns, blind alleys and dead ends; the labyrinth is a circular path that has one through route and is not designed to be difficult to navigate. The requirement of the labyrinth is that one has a willing and receptive mind-set to keep following the path to the center and engage in the experience as it unfolds.

The journey of the labyrinth can be thought of as a symbolic pilgrimage, as a metaphor for our life's journey. A labyrinth is an archetype with which we can have a direct experience. At its deepest level, the labyrinth is a pictogram representing a journey to the center of our deepest self, then back out into the world with a broadened understanding of who we are.

When one walks a labyrinth, one starts on the outskirts, follows a specified path that circles around and, in an ordered fashion, comes closer and closer to the center. The labyrinth is designed to teach us about ourselves through our journey inward. Although the outer paths seem pedestrian, they are necessary to create a foundation and make the journey to the center more meaningful. In the same way, we can learn about the power of transformation by acknowledging and developing our internal selves and intentionally cultivating higher internal experience. Looking inward changes us.

This book is divided into two parts, and so begins our labyrinth. Again, the outer paths prepare us for the journey ahead. Broadly, part one examines selected subject matter in neuroscience, biochemistry, and neurocardiology that involves emotion.

In the initial stages of part one—and on the outskirts of our journey—we begin by defining and differentiating the concept of stress and its associated terms. Understanding these distinctions is of primary importance in the examination of stress and anxiety; this understanding lays the groundwork necessary to grasp the subsequent and significant ramifications of the stress and anxiety response. Because stress and anxiety have become such household words and still defy a standard definition, it is important to have a working understanding of these concepts.

As we travel further into our labyrinth, we take a closer look at stress and anxiety, as these are what prevent us from living in an internally calm, peaceful, and loving state. The stress response is a physiological and biochemical reality. We have all experienced it. Sometimes it is vague, and at other times it is debilitating and overpowering. Some people feel it as tension in their head, some as tightness in the chest, and some as outright panic. Stress prevents us from thinking clearly, from remembering things we know, from behaving in a loving manner. We may literally become addicted to it.

Accordingly, then, we examine the physiological, biochemical, and electro-cardiological implications of anxiety and the anxiety response. Major considerations are shared regarding the automatic and subconscious nature of fear and anxiety that are essential in understanding and transforming negative emotional reaction patterns. We explore the powerful impact of the anatomy of the brain, the way it processes anxiety and emotion, and the inadequacy of traditional stress management techniques that have overlooked this fundamental consideration.

Stress and anxiety perpetuate themselves. As one consistently exposes oneself to the biochemistry, cardiology, and neuroscience of stress and anxiety, profound physiological adaptations occur in the body and brain that perpetuate and exacerbate the stress cycle. We literally become more biologically capable of experiencing increased stress and begin to suffer increasing resultant negative effects from that stress. These negative effects can have profound implications for our health, our mental health, our relationships, and our lives.

Knowledge is power, and a working understanding of how our bodies react to stress and anxiety gives us a necessary picture of the grave damage we are doing to ourselves by the choices we make. The physiology, neuroscience, and biochemistry of stress and anxiety are profound and, left unchecked, perpetuate and create significant and detrimental changes in our bodies and our brains. The physiology, biochemistry, and perpetuating cycle of stress, the neuroscience of emotion, and the resultant adaptations in our bodies and psyches are important considerations. Our labyrinth is now gaining meaning.

As we voyage further through our labyrinth, we consider opposites. With an understanding of the tremendous negative consequences of stress and anxiety and the perpetuating nature of living from those states, we consider the reverse. Allowing ourselves to consistently experience positive, loving emotions not only profoundly changes the chemistry of our bodies, it facilitates important adaptations throughout our bodies and literally changes the structure and function of our brains.

As we begin to reverse the cyclic nature of stress and anxiety to one of calm and connection, we create a new, lower baseline of stress, and our bodies strive to establish this as the new state of equilibrium, or homeostasis. Prompted by fundamental changes in our biology, physiology, and biochemistry, we see improvements in our overall health and cognition, we perceive and react differently, our relationships change, and our perception of our world changes.

Allowing and training ourselves to consistently feel and experience positive and loving feelings changes the structure of our brain and the chemistry of our bodies. It changes the way we think, the way we act, the way we perceive our world, and the energy we generate and give back to it. Intentionally operating from positive feelings and higher emotions creates a systemwide cascade of biochemical and brain reaction patterns that profoundly affect our bodies, our brains, and those around us. The resiliency of the human spirit may quite literally be reflected in the human brain and the human body. Western science is beginning to validate what Wisdom traditions have espoused all along: Intentionally cultivating and experiencing internal peace, compassion, and gratitude changes our world.

At times, traveling a labyrinth may challenge us to look inside ourselves. The second part of this book encompasses what it takes for true transformation. True transformation is an experience, not just knowledge about something, and it must be incorporated into our daily lives. Sincerely reducing the stress and anxiety in our lives and looking inward must first be a choice, and then an experience. True transformation embraces the challenge of change and follows concrete steps for that change. Part 2 of this book takes the course of our labyrinth from knowledge to action.

In the initial stages of part two I present specific techniques to intentionally and routinely cultivate higher emotional states, complete with all the positive physiological adaptations consistent with those states. I call them *higher emotion and refocusing techniques,* or HEART, and I believe these practices are the most important information in this book.

Routine internal experience of any state will create the physiological and biological adaptations consistent with that state. These techniques were designed to intentionally cultivate routine internal experience of higher emotional states and, as a result, create measurable changes in our physiology, perceptions, behaviors, and lives.

Now at the center of our labyrinth and moving further into part two, we begin to assimilate the knowledge garnered in part one, and the experience of our lives, and examine the question of true willingness. Are you really ready to live differently? What do you have invested in "staying stuck"? How does the specific knowledge content of part one affect you, and what are concrete steps for effective change? How do you set a daily practice to internalize the information from part one and begin the process of genuine transformation? Do you, in truth, desire transformation? Do you have any fears about the process?

After presenting HEART and examining willingness, we consider concrete steps to reduce the stress and chaos in our lives and the changes we need to make in our personal lives to prepare us for deep change. I call this "tilling the soil." Like a gardener preparing to grow a vibrant crop, attention must be paid to a nurturing preparation and tilling the soil to prime for planting. If a gardener hastily plants a crop with no consideration for its readiness, the crop is most certainly doomed; conversely, the richer the soil is at planting, the more likely the new plant life will flourish. Tilling the soil for the purposes of this book involves identifying and taking concrete steps to reduce the stress and anxiety in our lives and to identify areas in our lives that, with a little attention, will allow us to thrive more successfully.

Change behavior theorists break change—or in our semantics, transformation—into specific and definable stages. Again, our working definition of transformation is taking action to move beyond our current form. The emphasis of this definition must be on action. It is my experience that most people desiring transformation never move beyond the contemplation or preparation stage, thus never taking effective action and by no means achieving true transformation. True transformation requires true willingness, converted into action.

Among some of the other topics covered in part two are tools and practices to successfully develop your inner compass and how to genuinely incorporate the neuroscience of emotional resilience in your daily life. Honoring the neuroscience of change means it won't happen without consistent experience and practice. The brain and its ingrained stress or negative patterns will not transform without regular alternative positive experience. Without that consistent and cultivated alternative experience, the information presented in part one will leave us stuck in our old patterns of living, even though we have the knowledge of how to live differently.

Everything we do and say affects our brains, our bodies, our lives, and our hearts. In essence, it becomes who we are. How do we recognize what is positive for us? How do we recognize what is negative for us? How do we create a "positive energy diet"? Additional topics covered in part two include recognizing and honoring drains to our personal energy and, conversely, enhancing situations that infuse our personal energy. Transformation is not a destination, but a journey, so we also address how to create situations for continual growth and how our subjective interpretation of events quite often determines their outcome.

The power of semantics, or the words we choose to use ascribe meaning, are a powerful determinant of our "emotional diet." Some argue that all words carry a positive or negative connotation by the way they are used or phrased, and that positive or negative energy directly affects those using the language as well as those exposed to the language. Semantics is explored in relation to our personal energy, our emotional reaction patterns, and our relationship to others. The words we say, the emotional tone we create, and the things we expose ourselves to all create brain and biochemical reaction patterns that enhance or diminish our lives. How do we, on an intentional and routine basis, cultivate circumstances in our lives to enhance positive semantics and positive energy exposure?

This book is about looking inward to find peace, to find our inner radiance, or inexhaustible source of wisdom, wealth, and power. It also documents how, by constantly and consistently experiencing the feeling states of higher emotion, we create measurable changes in our bodies and brains that profoundly affect our lives and the lives of those around us. As we journey out from the center of our labyrinth, we honor our own uniqueness. We understand that at our core is a radiance entirely ours. To truly honor who we are, we need to honor this uniqueness, celebrate who we are meant to be, follow the paths that are prompted by this guidance, and bring our unique gifts into our lived experience.

The Importance of Reflective Writing

As the topic of authentic willingness for transformation reappears many times throughout this book, some of the practices incorporated here challenge the reader to take the journey from cognitive knowledge to the lived experience of sincere transformation through action. One of the most significant of these practices is completing the reflection exercises presented throughout the book. In completing the reflection exercises, the reader is challenged to routinely take the abstract concepts being presented and reflect, personalize, and process at a much deeper level than would be attained by merely reading the material. Although the tendency may be to skip the reflection exercises, this is a great mistake because these exercises are a large part of what facilitates the passage from knowledge, through experience and action, to foundational change.

Reflective writing, more than many other activities, helps facilitate the process of cultivating internal peace. There is evidence that this is true because personal writing calls upon both the right and left temporal lobes of the brain. What is significant about this process is that our "speaking self" is believed to be on the surface of the left temporal lobe and is responsible for the constant inner monologue that sometimes obscures our "silent self." Many researchers believe there is a mirror spot on the right temporal lobe that is responsible for what we experience as our silent self, the part of our brain that brings our feelings into awareness.

Because reflective writing connects these two areas, all at once our constant inner chatter seems to be quieted, as we bring our deeper feelings to conscious awareness. Our sense of our internal self is more accessible and made more apparent. When our sense of internal self is made more apparent, we are better able to connect to what we intuitively know to be true, and we can live more congruently with that self, thus further reducing the stress, chaos, and anxiety in our lives. Additionally, reflective writing gives us insight and guidance for further cultivation of our internal selves and the power that comes from living from that state.

Life is experience, not just knowledge about how to live. An important culmination to the labyrinth experience is the authentic integration of what we bring back from our journey inward and incorporate into our lived experience. "Putting it together" is the development of an action plan examining what it was that most resonated with us in our journey inward, along with concrete plans on how to incorporate those truths into our daily existence.

My friend Jeannie Huber tells me the story of many rabbis jointly philosophizing about Moses coming down from the mountain and what it would have been in God's voice that made Moses recognize it, deeply believe it, and recognize that the message he got was something he needed to bring back to humanity. He needed to recognize that voice as the voice of God and yet not as separate from himself. After much debate and exploration, the answer that they came up with was that the voice that Moses heard must have been in his own likeness.

This book is about intentionally cultivating a state of reduced stress and anxiety, through which we transform our bodies, brains, and minds by consistently practicing emotional refocusing and fostering states of internal peace and higher internal experience. Developing those states can transform our lives. This book attempts to facilitate that process by synthesizing some of the wonderful scientific information in the fields of neuroscience, psychophysiology, and biochemistry to help put it in a truly applicable form and examine some hard issues inhibiting true transformation.

No change or adaptation will occur in our bodies, relationships, or lives by merely learning about these concepts without true, cultivated, and consistent experience. Application and experience are the crucial ingredients. This book offers some avenues, backed by scientific evidence, to begin the transformative process. The most important of these is routine practice of the higher emotion and refocusing techniques, or HEART. Moreover, authentically engaging in the journal activities and reflective writing exercises are of foundational importance, as these activities help us access our internal selves and facilitate true transformation.

The process proposed here takes courage, willingness, sincere engagement, and a genuine desire for transformation. It is possible to live a life of greatly reduced stress and anxiety, a life where our bodies and brains transform from positive emotion, and a life centered in clear awareness of our interconnection to that which is ineffable.

This book is written with the intention of being understandable to the reader. I have done my best to take important scientific concepts and present them in a coherent, clear, and comprehensible way. The science of stress and anxiety and the science of intentionally cultivating higher emotional states needs to voyage out of the exclusiveness of science and into the understanding and practice of the human experience.

To reduce the chaos in our lives, we must first reduce the chaos within ourselves. To repattern our lives to function optimally, from a state of emotional ease, we must first repattern our brains and bodies to function from that state. To have lives based on calm, coherence, and love, we must first have calm, coherence, and love within ourselves and take concrete steps to integrate our newly developed internal experience to our outward existence.

The challenge of the labyrinth is not to navigate the proposed path as it is with a maze; the real challenge of the labyrinth is to have the courage to begin the journey inward.

REFERENCES

1. Dyer, W., *Your Sacred Self: Making the Decision to be Free* (New York: Harper Collins, 1995).

2. Astin, A. W., "Why Spirituality Deserves a Central Place in Liberal Education," *Liberal Education* 90:2 (2004): 34–41.

3. Lindholm, J. A., and H. S. Astin, "Understanding the 'Interior' Life of Faculty: How Important is Spirituality?" *Religion and Education* 33:2 (2006): 64–90.

4. Astin, "Why Spirituality Deserves."

5. Das, L. S., *Awakening the Buddha Within: Tibetan Wisdom for the Western World* (New York: Broadway Books, 1997).

6. Dyer, W., *The Power of Intention: Learning to Co-Create Your World Your Way* (Carlsbad, CA: Hay House, 2004).

7. Lindholm, J. A., "The 'Interior' Lives of American College Students: Preliminary Findings from a National Study," in *Passing on the Faith: Transforming Traditions for the Next Generation of Jews, Christians, and Muslims,* ed. J. L. Heft (New York: Fordham University Press, 2006): 75–102.

8. Joseph, R., *Neurotheology* (San Jose, CA: University Press, 2002).

9. LeDoux, J., *Synaptic Self: How Our Brains Become Who We Are* (New York: Penguin, 2002).

10. Damasio, A., *The Feeling of What Happens: Body and Emotions in the Making of Consciousness* (San Diego, CA: Harcourt, 1999).

11. Begley, S., *Train Your Mind, Change Your Brain: How a New Science Reveals Our Extraordinary Potential to Transform Our Lives* (New York: Ballantine Books, 2007).

12. Lipton, B., *The Biology of Belief: Unleashing the Power of Consciousness, Matter and Miracles* (Santa Rosa, CA: Elite Books, 2005).

13. Moore, T., *Care of the Soul: A Guide for Cultivating Depth and Sacredness in Everyday Life* (New York: HarperCollins, 1992).

14. Gallup, G. H., "Remarkable Surge of Interest in Spiritual Growth Noted as Next Century Approaches," *Emerging Trends* 12:1 (1998): 3–5.

15. Hicks, E., and J. Hicks, *Ask and It Is Given: Learning to Manifest Your Desires* (Carlsbad, CA: Hay House, 2004).

16. Pert, C., *Molecules of Emotion: The Science behind Mind–Body Medicine* (New York: Scribner, 1997).

17. McCraty, R., and M. Atkinson, "The Effect of Emotions on Short-Term Heart Rate Variability Using Power Spectrum Analysis," *American Journal of Cardiology* 76:14 (1995): 1089–1093.

18. Covey, Stephen R., A. Roger Merrill, Rebecca R. Merrill, *First Things First: To Live, to Love, to Learn, to Leave a Legacy* (New York: Simon & Schuster, 1994).

19. Ornish, D., *Dean Ornish's Program for Reversing Heart Disease* (New York: Ballantine, 1990).

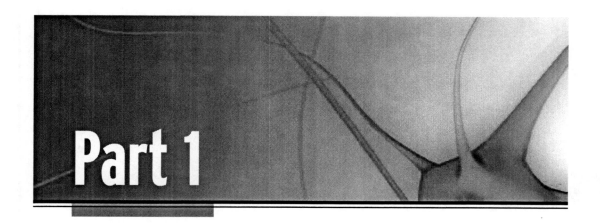

Part 1

Physiological Foundations of Negative and Positive Internal Experience

CHAPTER two

Stress, Chaos, and Anxiety

Introduction: What Is Stress?

In my opinion—and I have substantial physiological evidence to back it up—feelings of stress, chaos, anxiety, hate, anger, and fear are the most common obstacles to a higher internal experience. As we progress through the initial stages of our metaphorical labyrinth to the transformative process presented in this book, we will differentiate between the profound physiological implications and adaptations we experience as a result of lower emotional states as opposed to higher emotional states. We will also take a scientific look at how the intentional cultivation of higher emotional states can lead to higher internal states, higher potential, greater productivity, and possibly even higher states of consciousness. First, however, we must begin with a clear concept of what stress is and why it is so damaging to our emotional health, physical health, and level of internal experience. These are the outer paths of the labyrinth. In and of themselves they may seem pedestrian, but they are necessary to build the important knowledge foundation from which to build.

Stress, anxiety, and internal chaos, by their very definition, cut us off from our internal self or feelings of internal peace. We usually think of stress as coming from an externally chaotic life, but in rare instances, we see people who function peacefully among the chaos. Conversely, we see others who would seem to lead a stress-free life but are wracked by internal stress, depression, or anxiety. Understanding what stress and anxiety are and how those states correlate with the condition of our internal experience is crucial if we are to live calm, peaceful, and productive lives.

What is stress? When I ask that question in my stress management classes, I typically get myriad answers. Some cite work, relationships, bills, schoolwork, exhaustion, and just trying to survive. Others focus on feeling as if they are being pulled in many directions, feeling overwhelmed, feeling that there is never enough time, or struggling to live up to personal or external expectations. Still others describe feelings of free-floating anxiety, fear, depression, a psychological burden of internal issues, or physical manifestations commonly associated with stress, including headaches, frustration, fatigue, and strain.

Though I have posed this question to hundreds of university students and students of life, a definitive answer eludes us. Yet, there is no doubt that everyone knows exactly what stress is because they have experienced it, because they have *felt* it. We may not have adequate words to describe it, but from a feeling state we know it well. We have felt the emotional unease or discomfort that accompanies stress, anxiety, depression, and internal chaos.

When I tell people I meet that I teach stress management, they often respond with an audible and physical sign of relating to the feeling of stress. Many people make an off-handed comment that they should take the class, whether they are a student at the university or not. They want to talk further because they desperately want an answer, a solution to the disabling anxiety they feel. Many students tell me that the class is in such high demand that they try for years to enroll and often can't gain acceptance until the quarter before they graduate—if they are lucky. The demand for a solution to stress and anxiety is pervasive, but a clear-cut definition of exactly what it is remains elusive.

In Chapter One I introduced the term *ineffable*, referring to feeling states that cannot be adequately described in words. Ineffable may also be used to describe stress. We may use words that describe the things that stress us out, the general feeling of being overwhelmed and exhausted, or the physical manifestation of stress, but the words and descriptions fall short of the reality of the feeling state of stress. The truth is that we know stress, anxiety, and depression because we feel them. They create a powerful negative internal experience, and we feel the disconnect from the peace and productivity of our internal selves.

The inability to sufficiently describe the depth of feeling of stress or anxiety may stem from differences in the origination points in the brain between cognitive or conscious descriptions and the emotion of feeling. In other words, reasoning through word descriptions is associated with a very different place in the brain than where emotions are originally felt and activated. It's like trying to use words to convey the essence of deep and sincere love. Something important gets lost in the transition from feeling it to describing it.

Stress is a powerful feeling of emotional unease generated in the limbic system, the emotional center of the brain, and processed by the right temporal lobe. A spot on the left temporal lobe is the source of establishing words to describe the feeling. Somewhere in the transition, the depth of the debilitating effects is diminished, although the feeling is not. We may not always be able to accurately associate words to the feelings, but we cannot, and must not, deny the feeling and deleterious effects it causes in our lives or our ability to live optimally.

Working definitions of the different aspects and associated terms of stress are shared later in this chapter. At this point it is important to clarify that I use the term *stress* as an all-encompassing feeling of emotional unease, or dis-ease. Stress may take the form of a free-floating anxiety, a feeling of depression, a feeling of being emotionally or psychologically paralyzed or disabled, or a feeling of being internally chaotic or pressured. The feeling of stress may also take the form of an invisible barrier to growth. Sometimes we don't feel necessarily stressed, as we commonly interpret the term, but we just can't seem to get our lives on the track we want to be taking.

The Mind/Body Connection

These states are most often described as an internal feeling state. They can be accurately described as one in which internal peace and connection are decidedly absent. Having a concept of the feeling aspect of stress, anxiety, fear, or emotional reactive states is fundamental in understanding how to reduce their presence in our lives and how stress prevents us from living the lives we were meant to live.

A substantial body of contemporary research indicates that the quality and state of our being at any moment of awareness is rooted in the underlying state of our physiological and biochemical processes. More simply, what is going on in our minds and souls is reflected in our bodies, and what is going on in our bodies is reflected in our minds and souls. Neuroscientist Antonio Damasio states:

> . . . there are organism states in which the regulation of life processes becomes efficient, or even optimal, free-flowing and easy. This is a well-established physiological fact. It is not a hypothesis. The feelings that usually accompany such physiologically conducive states are deemed "positive," characterized not just by absence of pain but by varieties of pleasure. There also are organism states in which life processes struggle for balance and can even be chaotically out of control. The feelings that usually accompany such states are deemed "negative," characterized not just by absence of pleasure but by varieties of pain.[1]

Damasio goes on to state, "The fact that we, sentient and sophisticated creatures, call certain feelings positive and other feelings negative is directly related to the fluidity or strain of the life process."[2] The essence of his idea is that we call certain emotional feelings "positive" and others "negative" because these experiences directly reflect the physiological and psychological impact on the body.

When we experience stress, depression, or anxiety, we are in internal chaos. The constant static of those states, like the static of a radio receiver, blocks us from tuning in to who we are at the deepest level, and it seems we can't even get in touch with what we know to be fundamentally true. When we are in these states, we are not physiologically or biochemically capable of achieving what has been commonly described as the "flow state," being in the "zone," or in the terms of this book, achieving a higher internal experience. We live and perform our best when we are internally coherent.

In *The Spontaneous Fulfillment of Desire*, Deepak Chopra calls this state of internal coherence the *synchronicity* of the body. He describes synchronicity as a state where our internal processes are in sync and we are in touch with our internal reference point. Chopra asserts that developing this synchronicity is a means of getting in touch with our internal selves, a path to meaning and purpose in our lives. He also makes a strong point that if we are stressed, we can't even begin to think about developing synchronicity of the body.[3] A body in chaos from stress is in direct physiological opposition to a positive internal experience.

The concept that negative feelings reflect physiological states that are out of balance and may even be chaotically out of control will be revisited on many different levels throughout this book. There is substantial evidence that these internally chaotic states are reflected in our biochemistry, that the neurohormones and neuropeptides produced and released throughout our body through a myriad of negative emotional reactions may potentially affect every cell in our body.[4] Other substantial research indicates the electrophysiological patterns emanating from our hearts' electrical activity reflect a different pattern whether we are internally coherent or suffering from frustration, stress, anxiety, or emotional unease.[5]

Also of importance is the research by Bruce Lipton that challenges the long-held assumption that genes alone control our biology. As will be shared later in this book, his work documents the fact that genes are often activated, or not activated, by what is going on biochemically and energetically in our bodies as a result of the thoughts and feelings we display every day. Finally, recent and convincing research on the neuroplasticity of the brain—that is, the brain's ability to change according to the circumstances to which it is exposed—indicates that we literally have the capacity to rewire the neural connections in our brains, dependent on our consistently experienced emotional state, whether that state is positive or negative.

The body is extremely adaptable. What we constantly and consistently expose it to, it will assume, through physiological changes, as its primary operating pattern. If we expose our bodies to stress, anxiety, and emotional unease, we literally train our bodies to experience more of the same. Additionally, if we are developing our bodies and brains to consistently operate from a state of stress, anxiety, and emotional unease, we are unknowingly preventing ourselves from creating a state conducive to internal coherence, higher internal experience, or physiological synchronicity. In other words, we are creating and living from chaotic physiological states that block the path to our productive internal experience and to meaning and purpose in our lives.

The physiology and biochemistry of stress, anxiety, and emotional unease are profound and leave little room for internal development, or internal peace; for the biological impact of these two states are in direct opposition to each other.

Concepts of Stress and Anxiety

To gain a deeper understanding of what stress is, and consequently what steps to take to reduce that stress, it is necessary to explore some of its associated components and terms. Though the terms *stress* and *anxiety* may seem vague and hard to define, these feeling states are deeply and frequently felt.

Formal definitions of stress are frequently as varied and vague as people's personal experiences with it. However, the physiological and biological implications of stress and anxiety are very real. Research on the causes and impact in the area of stress, and scientific discussion of the concept of stress are varied. Because of the numerous ways stress has been defined and examined in research, it must be considered "a general or collective term that encompasses many applications."[6] To put it more simply, stress is everywhere, and the term is used differently in different contexts.

Stress is often used as a reference to a specific stressor, the internal feelings of stress, tension or anxiety caused by that stressor, or the biological responses resulting from a person's perception of that stressor.[7] Is stress merely something that causes us to feel uneasy? Could it refer less to the things that cause us stress and more to our reaction to those things? Is it the biological impact of our reaction to those things? Is it the long-term consequences of exposure?

To gain an understanding of the detrimental physiological, biochemical, and cognitive effects of stress and anxiety and the positive physiological, biochemical, and cognitive effects of emotional resilience, we first must be completely clear about what we're experiencing. Thus, we must first clarify and differentiate between the terms often associated with these states to avoid confusion. These are all separate, but interconnected, concepts, and understanding the distinctions between the terms helps us understand the stress process as a whole, which is the first step in cultivating a state of internal peace and productivity.

Let's examine the terms *stress, stressor, homeostasis, stress response,* and *distress.* In addition to a description of these terms, I will include practical applications, with intent to make them "real" and reveal their importance in our lives. Also included is an in-depth discussion of the fear and anxiety response, because in that response we begin to comprehend the crucial dynamics of emotion, the importance of internal experience, and the power of knowledge and change.

Stress

This term defies easy definition. Many definitions and meanings have been ascribed to the term; however, general agreement is still lacking. One author states, "Attempts to define stress have always danced around a certain vagueness implicit in this term."[8] Again, we border on the ineffable, a word, that in itself, is beyond words.

An additional problem in ascribing a word description to the concept of stress is that some will assume a narrow description of the term and believe they don't match that description, even though they still feel a general sense of emotional unease, unhappiness, or separation of self. This manifestation of stress may be felt as a general feeling of dissatisfaction or an inability to grow or be productive in a way that feels internally coherent with who they are.

I would argue that *stress* is an all-encompassing state of emotional unease or discomfort rooted in biological processes, a state that blocks us from internal peace and higher internal experience.

The confusion surrounding the use of this term in research is that it has been simultaneously used to describe the stressful stimulus, or the things that stress us out; the adaptive responses, or how our bodies and psyches try to regain balance; and the negative physiological and psychological results of stress response.[9] However, researchers use the term generally to refer to a negative set of physiological and/or psychological characteristics. My underlying belief is that what is commonly characterized as stress is better defined as the internal experience of the anxiety response. When we begin to understand the dynamics of anxiety and the emotional reaction patterns in the brain, we can more clearly see why all of our traditional stress management tools have been only partially effective.

Evolution of the Term *Stress*

Hans Selye was the first person to use the term *stress* as we know it today. He described stress as a specific physiological reaction pattern and resultant adaptations by the body in response to some stimuli. In other words, something upsets the balance in our bodies, minds, or souls, and our bodies and psyches strive to regain that balance. Because he defined stress as the specific reaction pattern by the body in an attempt to rebalance itself after a disturbing force, he did not necessarily view stress as good or bad.

Selye did, however, define what he called the *General Adaptation Syndrome* or *Stress Syndrome*. Briefly, he described a set of physiological responses by the body as it attempts to return to the state of balance after exposure to some disturbing force. If these responses are inadequate in returning the body to balance because of inadequate, inappropriate, or excessive activation of compensatory responses, physical and psychological damage result.[10] The initial activation of these responses is often associated with emotional experiences such as anxiety, fear, or anger.[11]

What does all that mean in understandable and personally relevant terms? Our bodies, minds, and souls want and need to be in balance. When something is perceived to be a threat to that balance, we usually have some sort of negative emotional reaction, be it fear, anxiety, worry, or anger. Our psychophysiology—the combination of the body, mind, and soul—responds with a cascade of negative reaction patterns that consume us. Trying to compensate and regain its equilibrium, the body then kicks in with physical adaptations to regain that balance. Quite often, the disturbing force or forces are too great, last too long, or are repeated so that the body cannot regain the balance it desperately needs. It can't compensate for all the negative forces to which it is exposed, and the result is a physical and/or psychological breakdown.

Selye originally described stress as the process of the body trying to adapt and reestablish balance, but his description of the general adaptation or stress syndrome is what is usually accepted as stress. The word *syndrome* basically refers to a group of signs and symptoms that together are characteristic of a disease. Unresolved disturbing forces, either internally or externally perceived, leads to the breakdown of the body, mind, and soul.

Homeostasis, or "Balance"

Walter Cannon's contributions to the field of stress research center on the concept of homeostasis and how the body will strive to make physiological adaptations when that state of homeostasis is threatened. He describes the state of homeostasis as the "coordinated physiological reactions which maintain steady states of the body."[12] Translated from Greek, the term *homeostasis* means "steady or balanced state." Again, our bodies, minds, and souls desperately need to be in balance and will do everything they can do to reestablish balance when it is lost.

Cannon coined the phrase "flight or fight reaction," and he emphasized that the threat to homeostasis was often a result of the body's response to emotions. He also emphasized that homeostasis pertains not only to a steady state of physiological parameters, but also to states of mind. Cannon described a state of physiological and psychological equilibrium, or harmony. Homeostasis, then, is the "balanced, harmonious state of mind and body."[13] Our bodies, minds, and souls are one holistic functioning unit. This unit that is us strives for balance and craves harmony.

Perceived Stressor

Insel and Roth define the term *stressor* as "a physical or psychological event or condition that causes our body to elicit a physiological response, and disrupts our body's homeostasis."[14] Hales defines *stressors* as "the things that upset or excite us—whether they are positive or negative."[15] Although stressors can be perceived to be positive or negative, the term *stressor* is most frequently used to represent a negative or noxious stimulus.[16]

Put simply, stressors are the things that stress us out. A stressor may originate from external sources, such as perceived danger and difficult people or situations, or internal sources, such as thoughts, fears, anxiety, or negative emotions. Although they may originate externally or internally, the ultimate physical and emotional reaction is internal. In addition and maybe more importantly, many of us blame the stressor as the sole responsibility for the way we're feeling, when, in fact, it is a combination of our perception of the severity of that stressor and our own emotional reaction patterns. What is a stressor to me may not be a stressor to another person.

Stressors may be chronic, acute, or intermittent. This means they may be always present, as in time pressures, a difficult relationship, or work pressures; immediate and severe, as in the death of a loved one, a job loss, or the loss of an important relationship; or sometimes bothersome and sometimes not. In addition, the perception of the same stressor may elicit a varied physiological response among different people; thus, the ability of people to cope with the same stressor may be vastly different.[17] Again, it is the internal experience of the stressor that determines its severity.

According to Hubbard and Workman, the specific impact of a stressor on a person may be better explained by coexisting conditions, such as those involving strong emotions of love, fear, or anger.[18] In other words, when we have a stressor that is also connected to strong emotional feelings, like love, worry, or fear, the impact of that stressor is exacerbated. This underscores the relationship of the stress response and emotion: Learning the dynamics of emotional origination and developing emotional resilience are essential.

Of fundamental importance when defining the term *stressor* is the concept that a stressor may be real or perceived, but our body's psychological and physiological reactions are identical.[19] I once saw a friend shake with anxiety and fear and pace around with her heart racing when she thought her son had gotten hit in the head by a pitch in a little league game. She literally was sweating and about to have a panic attack. The interesting aspect of this scenario was that it only looked as if he had been hit. He dropped to the ground to avoid the pitch, but his mother's stress reaction remained elevated for the next two hours as if he had been severely hurt. Her internal experience of the event did not match the external reality.

Our perceptions of life's events are vital in our ability to maintain emotional balance and centeredness. How much do we anticipate catastrophes that never occur? Our brain makes little distinction between what we imagine could go wrong and what really happens, complete with all the negative physiological and psychological reactions. Legitimate stressors need to be examined and reduced in our lives. Creating imaginary stressors through catastrophizing, worrying, or distorted perceptions only serves to intensify our stress response and create more negative perceptions.

Determining Our Stressors
EXERCISE AND REFLECTION #1

Following are three widely accepted scales to measure stress. These scales measure the stressors present in our lives or our perceptions of those stressors. Complete the following stress scales according to the directions of each. After you have finished, complete and process the questions in your own personal reflective writing.

Life Changes Scaling

To get a feel for the possible health impact of the various recent events or changes in your life, think back over the past year and circle the points listed for each of the events that you experienced during that time. Many of these will be somewhat subjective. Answer to the best of your ability. Add up your points. A total score of anywhere from about 250 to 500 or so would be considered a moderate amount of stress. If you scored higher than that, you may face increased risk of illness; if you scored lower, consider yourself fortunate.

Health

An injury of illness which:		Major change in eating habits	27
Kept you in bed a week or more, or sent you to the hospital	74	Major change in sleeping habits	26
		Major change in your usual type	
Was less serious than that	44	Or amount of recreation	28
Major dental work	26		

Work

Change to a new type of work	51	With persons under your supervision	35
Change in your work hours or conditions	35	Other work troubles	28
Change in your responsibilities:		Major business adjustment	60
More responsibilities	29	Retirement	52
Fewer responsibilities	21	Loss of job:	
Promotion	31	Laid off from work	68
Demotion	42	Fired from work	79
Transfer	32	Correspondence course to help you in your work	18
Troubles at work:			
With your boss	29		
With coworkers	35		

Personal and Social

Change in personal habits	26	Girlfriend or boyfriend problems	39
Beginning or ending school	38	Sexual difficulties	44
Change of school or college	35	"Falling out" of a close relationship	47
Change of political beliefs	24	An accident	48
Change of religious beliefs	29	Minor violation of law	20
Change in social activities	27	Being held in jail	75
Vacation trip	24	Death of a close friend	70
New, close personal relationship	37	Major decision about future	51
Engagement to marry	45	Major personal achievement	36

Home and Family

Major change in living conditions	42	Due to marriage	41
Change in residence:		For other reasons	45
Move within same town or city	25	Change in arguments with spouse	50
Move to a different town, city or state	47	In-law problems	38
Change in family get-togethers	25	Change in marital status of your parents:	
Major change in health or behavior of a family member	55	Divorce	59
Marriage	50	Remarriage	50
Pregnancy	67	Separation from spouse:	
Miscarriage or abortion	65	Due to work	53
Gain of a new family member:		Due to marital problems	76
Birth of a child	66	Divorce	96
Adoption of a child	65	Birth of a grandchild	43
A relative moving in with you	59	Death of a spouse	119
Spouse beginning or ending work	46	Death of other family member:	
Child leaving home:		Child	123
To attend college	41	Brother or sister	102
		Parent	100

Financial

Major change in finances:		Loss or damage of personal property	43
Increased income	38	Moderate purchase	20
Decreased income	60	Major purchase	37
Investment or credit difficulties	56	Foreclosure on a mortgage or loan	58

Daily Hassles and Stress

For each of the following experiences, indicate to what degree it has been a part of your life over the past month by writing in the appropriate number.

1 = not at all part of my life

2 = only slightly part of my life

3 = distinctly part of my life

4 = very much part of my life

_____ 1. Disliking your daily activities
_____ 2. Lack of privacy
_____ 3. Disliking your work
_____ 4. Ethnic or racial conflict
_____ 5. Conflicts with in-laws or boyfriend's/girlfriend's family
_____ 6. Being let down or disappointed by friends
_____ 7. Conflict with supervisor(s) at work
_____ 8. Social rejection
_____ 9. Too many things to do at once
_____ 10. Being taken for granted
_____ 11. Financial conflicts with family members
_____ 12. Having your trust betrayed by a friend
_____ 13. Separation from people you care about
_____ 14. Having your contributions overlooked
_____ 15. Struggling to meet your own standards of performance and accomplishment
_____ 16. Being taken advantage of
_____ 17. Not enough leisure time
_____ 18. Financial conflicts with friends or fellow workers
_____ 19. Struggling to meet other people's standards of performance and accomplishment
_____ 20. Having your actions misunderstood by others
_____ 21. Cash-flow difficulties
_____ 22. A lot of responsibilities
_____ 23. Dissatisfaction with work
_____ 24. Decisions about intimate relationships
_____ 25. Not enough time to meet your obligations
_____ 26. Dissatisfaction with your mathematical ability
_____ 27. Financial burdens
_____ 28. Lower evaluation of your work than you think you deserve
_____ 29. Experiencing high levels of noise
_____ 30. Adjustments to living with unrelated person(s) (e.g., roommate)
_____ 31. Conflicts with family member(s)
_____ 32. Finding your work too demanding
_____ 33. Conflicts with friends
_____ 34. Hard effort to get ahead
_____ 35. Trying to secure loan(s)
_____ 36. Getting "ripped off" or cheated in the purchase of goods

_____ 37. Dissatisfaction with your ability at written expression
_____ 38. Unwanted interruptions of your work
_____ 39. Social isolation
_____ 40. Being ignored
_____ 41. Dissatisfaction with your physical appearance
_____ 42. Unsatisfactory housing conditions
_____ 43. Finding work uninteresting
_____ 44. Failing to get money you expected
_____ 45. Gossip about someone you care about
_____ 46. Dissatisfaction with your physical fitness
_____ 47. Gossip about yourself
_____ 48. Difficulty dealing with modern technology
_____ 49. Car problems
_____ 50. Hard work to look after and maintain home

Scoring:
Add up your responses and find your total below.

Very High Stress	>136
High Stress	116–135
Average Stress	76–115
Low Stress	56–75
Very Low Stress	51–55

Time Stress Questionnaire

The following list describes time-related difficulties people sometimes experience. Please indicate how often each is a difficulty for you, using numbers shown.

0 = Seldom or never a difficulty for me

1 = Sometimes a difficulty for me

2 = Frequently a difficulty for me

_____ My time is directed by factors beyond my control
_____ Interruptions
_____ Chronic overload—more to do than time available
_____ Occasional overload
_____ Chronic underload—too little to do in time available
_____ Occasional underload
_____ Alternating periods of overload and underload
_____ Disorganization of my time
_____ Procrastination
_____ Separating home, school, and work
_____ Transition from work or school to home
_____ Finding time for regular exercise
_____ Finding time for daily periods of relaxation
_____ Finding time for friendships
_____ Finding time for family
_____ Finding time for vacations
_____ Easily bored
_____ Saying "yes" when I later wish I had said "no"
_____ Feeling overwhelmed by large tasks over an extended period of time
_____ Avoiding important tasks by frittering away time on less important ones
_____ Feeling compelled to assume responsibilities in groups
_____ Unable to delegate because no one to delegate to
_____ My perfectionism creates delays
_____ I tend to leave tasks unfinished
_____ I have difficulty living with unfinished tasks
_____ Too many projects going at one time
_____ Getting into time binds by trying to please others too often
_____ I tend to hurry even when it's not necessary
_____ Lose concentration while thinking about other things I have to do
_____ Not enough time alone
_____ Feel compelled to be punctual
_____ Pressure related to deadlines

Scoring:

0–9	Low difficulty with time-related stressors
10–19	Moderate difficulty with time-related stressors
20 or more	High difficulty with time-related stressors

Now go back and underline the five most significant time-related stressors for you. Identify two concrete strategies you can take to help relieve each of these key stressors.

Stressor 1: _____

    1. _____

    2. _____

Stressor 2: _____

    1. _____

    2. _____

Stressor 3: _____

    1. _____

    2. _____

Stressor 4: _____

    1. _____

    2. _____

Stressor 5: _____

    1. _____

    2. _____

Personal and Reflective Writing

The personal and reflective writing recommended in this book is intended to be a personal exploration of the subjects presented. Although questions are presented to direct your writing, they are not meant to be answered verbatim and without contemplation. Though the impulse may be to skip the reflective writing, this is a great mistake because this writing is a large part of what facilitates the passage from knowledge, through experience and action, to foundational change.

These exercises are designed to help you personalize and process at a much deeper level than would be attained by merely reading the material.

Reflective writing, more than many other activities, helps facilitate the process of cultivating internal peace. Use the questions provided as guidance, and take the time to process any pertinent information that may resonate with you and to explore any worthwhile direction it may take you.

Questions for Exploration

Do you feel these scales accurately reflected your stress levels? Why or why not?

Which scale most accurately reflected what you perceive your stress levels to be?

Were your stresses concentrated in one specific area? How much internal stress do you feel from that area?

Sometimes people feel a significant amount of stress from a specific issue(s) but rate low on the scales. If this is true for you, explore why.

Do you feel there were some important areas missing?

From your own personal opinion (not from the scales), what are they biggest issues in your life that cause you to feel internal stress?

How do you feel when you are faced with those stressors?

At this point it should be clear that stress is a very personal experience. What one person may experience as stress may be very different than what another experiences. The key is to understand what stress is and to understand that it is an internal experience, a feeling state of being. As we progress further in our examination of stress, we begin to examine the physical implications of the stress response, as the mind, body, and spirit cannot be separated.

The Stress Response

Measurable physiological effects from exposure to a stressor characterize the stress response.[20] The stress response is usually defined by observation of predictable responses in heart rate, blood pressure, stress hormones, alterations in the immune system, the pattern of heart rate variability, and other physiological parameters.[21] What this all means is when we feel stress, either from an external or internal source, our body has predictable responses. Our heart may race, our blood pressure may rise, we are flooded with cortisol and other stress hormones, and we may feel out of sync, get sick or worse.

Additionally, there may be pronounced cortical inhibition—that is, a person under stress may exhibit reduced cognitive functioning.[22] The cortex is considered the "thinking" part of the brain. Basically, pronounced cortical inhibition means we can't think; there is an obvious difference between this state and our normal thinking state. We have all been in situations in which we were so stressed that we momentarily couldn't think clearly, that we felt confused or went blank. This is due to cortical inhibition, and it is a physiological reality.

There's a physiological reason why we are unable to concentrate in situations that make us nervous, like taking an exam, giving a speech, or being involved in a car collision. When we experience stress, stress hormones flood our brain and reduce its thinking and reasoning capacity. Again, the stress response a person experiences may be profoundly affected by his or her coexisting emotional state or past experiences associated with a similar event.

Distress

Distress occurs when the "physiological and psychological compensatory mechanisms activated by the body's stress response fail to return the body to homeostasis."[23] It is usually associated with emotional experiences such as anxiety, worry, fear, or anger. Basically, distress is when our bodies and psyches begin to break down after becoming exhausted trying to regain balance. We have given ourselves more than we can handle, either internally or externally, psychologically or physically, or all of the above. *Webster's New World Concise Medical Dictionary* defines distress as "mental or physical suffering or anguish."[24] Suffering and anguish are strong terms. Suffering and anguish are not conducive to internal coherence or to a positive internal experience; they are associated with lower emotional states such as anxiety, worry, fear, and anger. Given this evidence, there seems to be a strong connection between the level of emotional experience and the level of physiological and psychological response.

Anxiety

According to *Newsweek* reporter Jennifer Ozols, anxiety disorders are now the most common form of mental illness among Americans. In her article "It's an Anxious Time," she reports that at least 19 million adults in the United States—more than 13 percent of the country's adult population—suffer from some form of disorder associated with anxiety. She also argues that in our current culture those numbers are likely to stay elevated or even increase.[25]

Anxiety is a specific form of stress, and understanding the process of the anxiety response in the brain begins to give us the necessary tools to reduce or minimize that response. As the result of an extensive and passionate search of the subject matter, I believe that understanding the anxiety response and further understanding how emotion is processed in the brain are the key to transformation. Furthermore, I believe replacing that anxiety response with internal calm, peace, connection, and productivity—essentially a higher internal experience—is the metal that forges that key.

The Anxiety Response

Part 2 of this book presents transformative techniques for developing emotional resilience, reducing the anxiety response, and cultivating our internal selves. But before we understand the significance of refocusing our emotional attention, we must have a basic understanding of the physiology of anxiety, fear, and negative emotion. Understanding the physiology and detrimental effects of anxiety, worry, fear, and other negative emotions leads us to a better understanding of how these processes work with positive loving emotions, as these two emotional states are in direct biochemical and neural opposition to each other.

Webster's New World Concise Medical Dictionary defines anxiety as "apprehension of danger or dread accompanied by restlessness, tension, tachycardia (elevated heart rate), and dyspnea (shortness of breath)."[26] Hales defines anxiety as "a feeling of apprehension and dread stemming from the anticipation of danger, and sometimes accompanied by physical symptoms which may cause significant distress and impairment to an individual."[27] Chrousos, Loriaux, and Gold describe anxiety as a psychological state characterized by feelings of impending danger.[28]

There is substantial consensus in the literature that anxiety is a state of apprehension often accompanied by a variety of physiological responses, including impaired cognitive functioning. In other words, we don't think as clearly as we should be able to, given the circumstances. Insel and Roth state that when dealing with anxiety, it is common to think less rationally than when we are calm.[29] There is also consensus in the literature that psychological stimuli in the form of fear and apprehension most often stimulate the anxiety response.[30]

Where does the fear come from? What causes this apprehension? Hubbard and Workman conceptualize anxiety as the body's response to an anticipated and feared future event; this response may be triggered by a significantly emotional past event.[31] In exploring the physiological and cognitive implications of anxiety, we must first examine how past negative experiences activate the feeling of anxiety, often without conscious thought. Following is a description of that process; first in academic terms and then in terms that may be more personally understandable or applicable.

At the center of the human brain is a "complicated web of ancient circuitry."[32] It is hyperreactive to perceived threats, a response that evolved long before the neocortex, which is responsible for conscious awareness. As a result, when this brain circuit functions independently, it may be beyond conscious thought. Joseph LeDoux of New York University calls this the "emotional brain" and asserts that it is highly attuned to signs of potential danger. Through a process called *fear conditioning*, LeDoux theorizes, this portion of the brain can learn to perceive a mundane stimulus as a warning sign.[33]

Cowley explains that deep inside our brains, within this complex circuitry, lies a small almond-shaped structure called the *amygdala*. The amygdala is responsible for storing subconscious emotional memory, and it plays a significant role in the activation of fear. It is considered the fear system's command center and, again, it is not part of the neocortex so it is not involved in conscious awareness. The amygdala is often activated as the body's first response to a perceived threat and immediately activates the body's physiological stress response.

By the time a perceived threat can be consciously controlled, the amygdala has already activated the body's stress response, and the body is experiencing a flood of biochemical and cardiovascular reactions. The amygdala is also storing this response deep in emotional memory.[34] Cowley clarifies:

> An activated amygdala doesn't wait around for instructions from the conscious mind. Once it perceives a threat, it can trigger a bodywide emergency response within milliseconds. Jolted by impulses from the amygdala, the nearby hypothalamus produces a hormone called corticotropin releasing factor, or CRF, which signals the pituitary and adrenal glands to flood the bloodstream with epinephrine (adrenaline), norepinephrine and cortisol. . . . The stress hormones also act on the brain, creating a state of heightened alertness and supercharging the circuitry involved in memory formation. The amygdala tells the rest of the brain, hey whatever happens, make a strong memory of it.[35]

Once it stores that stressful memory, the amygdala can be easily activated by the apprehension of a similar upcoming event. The same process can occur whether the event is extremely significant or a constant low-grade stimulation.[36] Emotional memories such as fear, apprehension, or anxiety can be triggered by an anticipated event similar to the past event, whether or not those emotions are appropriate for the current situation.[37] Additionally, the amygdala takes in a variety of impressions (e.g., sights, sounds, smells, facial expressions, perceptions of nonverbal behavior). It then looks for a match and triggers a systemwide physiological and psychological response, whether or not it is appropriate for that situation.[38]

When this perception reaches the prefrontal cortex of the brain, the emotional reaction may be tempered if it is deemed inappropriate; however, the initial physiological responses have already been activated. Furthermore, for people especially prone to anxiety, the prefrontal cortex may have a diminished capacity to control the amygdala, allowing it

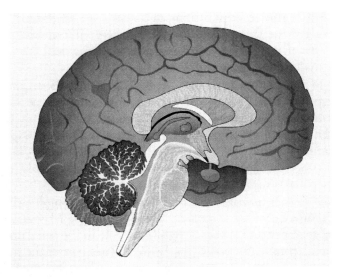

FIGURE 2.1 A diagram of the human brain, showing the difference in structure and location of the limbic system and neocortex.

to act unheeded and arouse fear in nonthreatening situations.[39] Additionally, recent research has shown that the teenage and young adult brain has a reduced prefrontal cortex and an amygdala that is more active than the fully formed adult brain, presumably making the teenage brain more prone to anxiety.[40]

A simple example of this process can be illustrated by a person with an intense fear of snakes who jumps in fear at the sight of a stick on the ground. The first emotional reaction is that the stick is a snake, and a whole series of biochemical and cardiovascular reactions are activated in that person's body before he has the chance to cognitively discern that the object is just a stick. Another example is that of a student getting ready to take an important exam. Her subconscious emotional reaction may be recalling past failures and sending anxious physiological reactions throughout her body, including cognitive impairment, without conscious awareness of this reaction.

How does this all work? Figure 2.1 demonstrates a basic side view of the inside of the human brain. The inner structure is what some researchers call the *limbic system*. The limbic system, which includes the amygdala, is thought of as the emotional part of the brain, which is very distinct from the neocortex, or thinking part of the brain. The neocortex is the area on the outside layers of the brain. Although information constantly travels back and forth between both parts of the brain, the neural connections leading from the limbic system to the neocortex are stronger and more numerous than those leading from the neocortex to the limbic system.

What this means is that information being processed by the limbic system (our emotional center) and sent to the neocortex (our thinking and reasoning center) is stronger and quicker than information going in the reverse direction. Fear, anxiety, and worry activated in the amygdala get a head start on our ability to temper that response with reason. Additionally, as we will explore in Chapter Four, the area of the brain that is richest in the production and use of our body's biochemicals is also the part of the brain that is involved in emotion.[41]

Three more fundamentally important points need to be made, after which I will do my best to synthesize and explain why this information is crucial in our transformative journey inward. Although these points are made separately, they are interconnected in function.

First, the emotional system can act independently of the neocortex, meaning that information reaching and being processed by the emotional center may or may not carry with it cognitive awareness. In other words, we may have an incredibly strong emotional reaction to something, a powerful feeling of physical and psychological unease without even knowing why. Even when the neocortex is involved, its ability to diminish a strong emotional reaction is limited. In other words, I can reason why I shouldn't feel a certain way, but I still feel that way.

I have a funny experience with this whole process. The amygdala is very sensitive to smells, sounds, and subconscious sights. I have a song that, for no apparent reason, makes me cry. It happens almost every time I hear it. It is a song from my childhood, yet I have no conscious memory of why the song elicits such a strong reaction. It has even become a joke with my children and me. We will be driving in the car, and I will put the song on the stereo just to prove to my kids that I can make it through listening to it without crying. I am wrong every time. I will start the whole process laughing and teasing, but invariably I am in tears by the end of the song—even if I am laughing and crying at the same time. I still have no conscious reason why.

Thus is the subconscious nature of many emotional or anxiety reaction patterns. Many times we don't even know why we are experiencing specific emotional states, especially ones filled with fear and anxiety, yet their response may be all consuming. Or, more often, our response to a stressor or stressful event evokes this anxiety reaction in us, and we automatically assume our response is due to the stressor or event that is currently happening.

This assumption leads to the second point: Information can go directly to the amygdala without conscious processing. What this means is that we don't even have to be consciously aware of the thing or things that are setting off our anxiety reaction. This can be illustrated by research done on something called *binocular rivalry*. When a person is presented with two images, one for each eye, the person visually perceives only one image at a time. For instance, if a person is looking through a pair of binoculars, but each eye piece displays a different image, the person can only see one image at a time. Although the image that is consciously seen may be pleasant, and the one unseen may be disturbing, the amygdala can respond to the image that is beyond conscious awareness.

To add to this example, other research shows the amygdala can respond to either pleasant or disturbing facial images flashed so fast on a computer they are beyond conscious awareness. To underscore this concept, when the amygdala is activated, we feel that reaction as whole body emotional or feeling reaction. It is natural to want to attribute the emotional feeling reaction to what we are consciously aware of—the situation "in front of our face"—whether that situation warrants that degree of emotional reaction or not. Most of the time, it does not.

Chapters 8 and 9 present tools for developing emotional resilience. The first step is to notice your physical reaction when you are experiencing stress or anxiety. If you have a noticeable physical reaction, most likely this response is being initiated by the amygdala, and it had more to do with stored unconscious emotional reaction patterns than what is currently going on in your current circumstance. Realizing that this reaction comes from unconscious stored emotional reaction patterns is the first step to diffusing those patterns.

Two examples of this subconscious emotional reaction pattern may be in subliminal advertising and immediately liking or disliking a person. In subliminal advertising an image is flashed so fast on a movie, TV, or computer screen that it is beyond conscious awareness although it still elicits an emotional reaction. Subliminal advertising is controversial and many question its impact, but consider this example: You are watching TV late at night, feeling depressed and lonely. You have no idea why, but you suddenly feel a chocolate doughnut is the only thing that will make you feel emotionally comforted and secure.

There are likely other explanations for why you immediately like or dislike a person you meet for the first time, but this phenomenon can be an example of a subconscious emotional reaction. Although you may not be consciously aware of the likeness, this person may carry attributes that remind you of someone else. You may not make the connection consciously, but your amygdala may be activated and release an immediate emotional feeling of ease or unease. You may become consciously aware of the feeling activated in you, but not its initial cause.

This concept happens over and over again in relationships. For those who have had difficult relationships in the past with significant others, parents, siblings, classmates, or coworkers, for example, a facial expression, attitude, or situation in an entirely new relationship may set off an anxiety-filled reaction pattern. We, of course, feel the reaction and assume the circumstance we are currently in warrants that emotional reaction.

The third important point about the power of amygdala activation is that the initial trigger can also be subconscious. Figure 2.2 is an interpretation of how anxiety is stored and activated in our brains. Anxiety is a type of emotional memory, but it is not necessarily cognitive memory, or a memory of which we are consciously aware. Emotional memory is really a physiological, or physical, reaction in which we "feel" a specific emotional state throughout our body. Emotional memory, then, is the feeling state of physical and psychological unease associated with a conscious or subconscious reaction.

In the uppermost box in Figure 2.2, we see a negative perception of a stressor. That negative perception of a stressor leads to a psychological and physiological stress response throughout our body. Part of what happens through the physical release of stress hormones is that some of those hormones are carried by the vagus nerve straight to the amygdala to imprint the emotional memory. The next time we encounter anything that remotely matches that experience, our feeling or emotional responses are triggered.

Figure 2.2 is a simple representation. Because of the complex and circular nature of this response pattern, new information is stored continually. What is important about this third point regarding emotional memory storage and activation is that the initial trigger can be subconscious. We may not be consciously aware of the initial triggers, we may not even know why we have them in the first place, but we know them because we can feel them.

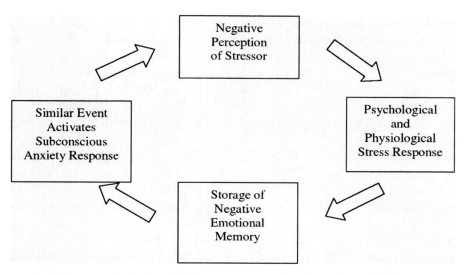

FIGURE 2.2   A conceptualization of the response cycle leading to anxiety.

The feeling aspect is all-important. Because we can feel the response to the triggers, this is the first key to be able to diffuse those triggers. If we do not understand how this whole process takes place, our initial impulse is to feel the feelings activated by this process and rationalize why we should feel this way given our current set of circumstances. If we are aware of this process, we can take notice of our triggers, understand that those triggers are coming as a result of stored emotional memory, disengage from the feeling reaction state in our body, and see the situation and our response more rationally.

The thread connecting all of these concepts is that, quite often, emotional reactions originate in a subconscious area of the brain. Even when they are brought to conscious awareness and cognitively processed, the impact of the emotional reaction can remain. The amygdala can react and send raw feelings of emotional reactions throughout our bodies, independent from and prior to rational thought.[42] They can be initially activated by something we are not even consciously aware of, yet the feeling we experience is very real. Many times, these processes work in concert.

Recall the story about my friend and her son at the little league game. She may not know why she has such a strong reaction of anxiety to any threat to the health of her children. Certainly, we all have fears and concerns about the health of our loved ones, but her response was so immediate and strong that she was not able to calm herself for hours. Let's interpret this story from the standpoint of the amygdala.

My friend's son is up to bat. Somewhere in her amygdala she has stored extreme anxiety regarding accidents; she has no conscious memory of why. As her son stands in for the pitch, she sees the ball hit his helmet, and he immediately drops to the ground. In reality, the ball has barely nicked his helmet. He instinctively drops to the ground to avoid getting hit. He gets up, dusts himself off, and trots down to first base.

However, his mother is still coping with her emotional reaction, independent of conscious thought, that he has been seriously injured. Her heart races and she shakes with fear. Her breathing is rapid, and she begins to sweat and pace. Even though she can see him standing on first base with a wide smile on his face, she cannot calm down. Her mind continues to focus on the catastrophe that could have been, which only intensifies her emotional and physiological reactions. In short, she is caught up in the circular nature of negative emotional reactive patterns, even though the reality of the situation does not warrant those reactions.

Understanding the anxiety response is crucial in comprehending its tremendous impact on our emotional reaction patterns and the way we feel at any given moment. Even when we are aware of these triggers, if we don't really "get" the process of what is happening in our brains, the information will not be as transformative as it could be. Noticing the feeling of stress or anxiety and recognizing that feeling as part of our inborn process are the first steps to diffusing that process.

The impact of habitual states of anxiety on interpersonal relationships and self-concept may be of great consequence. Research has shown that habitually experiencing some specific biochemical states—for example, the release of stress-induced hormones such as cortisol—actually increases the number of brain receptor sites for those chemicals and makes us more physiologically capable of perpetuating and increasing those stress-induced states.[43] Research has also shown that routine low-level "cortisol baths" significantly contribute to the development and onset of depression.[44]

Anxiety and distress are physiological, biochemical, and cognitive realities; we feel their effects all throughout our bodies and minds. The physiological effects of negative feelings play a part in reduced cognition, impaired reasoning, and more perceived stress, as well as damaged relationships, reduced self-concepts, and depression. In other words, we can't think, we feel overwhelmed, and we don't feel good about ourselves or anyone else.

Routinely noticing our specific triggers or feeling reaction patterns and replacing these negative physiological responses and adaptations with those generated by higher emotional states can have profound implications and possibilities for transformation. It can change how we live our lives. Routinely experiencing an intentional shift to a positive emotional state has been shown to literally rewire our brains, change the electrical patterns of our hearts, change the chemical composition of our bodies, and influence our genetic activation.

The process of emotional reaction patterns involving specific forms of negative emotion—namely, anxiety, fear, and worry—will be revisited in Chapter Five. It is very difficult to separate the discussion of anxiety from the larger discussion of emotion; however, due to the linear fashion of this book, I must do so. That's why we return to these concepts in Chapter Five, in greater depth, which will lead us to the power of turning inward to routinely experience the transformative power of gratitude, peace, calm, and loving kindness.

In Chapter Three, we will delve into the stress process and specific research in the area of stress. Chapter Four will include an activity associating stressful or happy events and our feeling states, along with an in-depth description of groups of people coming to this realization.

REFERENCES

1. Damasio, A., *Looking for Spinoza: Joy, Sorrow, and the Feeling Brain* (Orlando: Harcourt, 2003): p. 131.

2. Damasio, *Looking for Spinoza*, p. 131.

3. Chopra, D., *The Spontaneous Fulfillment of Desire: Harnessing the Infinite Power of Coincidence* (New York: Harmony, 2003).

4. Pert, C., *Molecules of Emotion: The Science Behind Mind–Body Medicine* (New York: Scribner, 1997).

5. McCraty, R., and M. Atkinson, "The Effect of Emotions on Short-Term Heart Rate Variability Using Power Spectrum Analysis," *American Journal of Cardiology* 76:14 (1995): 1089–1093.

6. Hubbard, J. R., and E. A. Workman, ed., *The Handbook of Stress: An Organ System Approach* (New York: CRC Press, 1998).

7. Chrousos, G. P., D. L. Loriaux, and P. W. Gold, "Mechanisms of Physical and Emotional Stress," in *Advances in Experimental Medicine and Biology*, Vol. 245, ed. National Institutes of Health (New York: Plenum Press, 1988).

8. Rosenzweig, M., A. L. Leiman, and S. M. Breedlove, *Biological Psychology: An Introduction to Behavioral, Cognitive, and Clinical Neuroscience*, 2nd ed. (Sunderland, MA: Sinauer Associates, 1999).

9. Ibid.

10. Chrousos, Loriaux, and Gold, "Mechanisms of Physical and Emotional Stress."

11. McCraty and Atkinson, "Effect of Emotions."

12. Chrousos, Loriaux, and Gold, "Mechanisms of Physical and Emotional Stress," p. 4.

13. Ibid.

14. Insel, P., and W. Roth, *Core Concepts in Health*, 4th ed. (Mountain View, CA: Mayfield, 2003).

15. Hales, D., *An Invitation to Health*, 10th ed. (Belmont, CA: Wadsworth, 2003).

16. Hubbard and Workman, *Handbook of Stress*.

17. Ibid.

18. Ibid.

19. Cowley, G., "Our Bodies, Our Fears," in special edition on Anxiety and Our Brain, *Newsweek*, February 24, 2003, 44–49.

20. Hubbard and Workman, *Handbook of Stress*.

21. Hubbard and Workman, *Handbook of Stress*; McCraty and Atkinson, "Effect of Emotions"; Rein, G., M. Atkinson, and R. McCraty, "The Physiological and Psychological Effects of Compassion and Anger," *Journal of Advancement in Medicine*, 8:2 (1995): 87–105.

22. Cowley, "Our Bodies, Our Fears"; Roozendaal, B., "Stress and Memory: Opposing Effects of Glucocorticoids on Memory Consolidation and Memory Retrieval," *Neurobiology of Learning and Memory* 78 (2002): 578–595; Rosenzweig, Leiman, Breedlove, *Biological Psychology.*

23. Chrousos, Loriaux, and Gold, "Mechanisms of Physical and Emotional Stress," p. 4.

24. Hensyl, W. R., ed. *Webster's New World/Stedman's Concise Medical Dictionary* (New York: Simon and Schuster, 1987).

25. Ozols, J., "It's an Anxious Time," *Newsweek,* December 1, 2004.

26. Hensyl, *Webster's New World.*

27. Hales, *Invitation to Health.*

28. Chrousos, Loriaux, and Gold, "Mechanisms of Physical and Emotional Stress."

29. Insel and Roth, *Core Concepts in Health.*

30. Hales, *Invitation to Health;* Hubbard and Workman, *Handbook of Stress;* Insel and Roth, *Core Concepts in Health.*

31. Hubbard and Workman, *Handbook of Stress.*

32. Cowley, "Our Bodies, Our Fears," p. 45.

33. LeDoux, J., *The Emotional Brain: The Mysterious Underpinnings of Emotional Life* (New York: Simon and Schuster, 1996).

34. Ibid.

35. Cowley, "Our Bodies, Our Fears," p. 46.

36. Ibid.

37. LeDoux, *Emotional Brain.*

38. Ibid.

39. Rosenzweig, Leiman, and Breedlove, *Biological Psychology.*

40. National Institute of Health, *Teenage Brain: A Work in Progress* (Bethesda, MD: Author, 2001).

41. Pert, *Molecules of Emotion.*

42. Goleman, D., *Emotional Intelligence: Why It Can Matter More than I.Q.* (New York: Bantam, 1994).

43. Rosenzweig, Leiman, and Breedlove, *Biological Psychology.*

44. National Institute of Mental Health, *Cognitive Research at the National Institute of Mental Health* (Bethesda, MD: Author, 2000).

CHAPTER three

The Stress Process

Introduction

The focus of this chapter is on the physiology of the stress process and the overall effects of stress on emotion and cognition. We will examine how the "feeling" states of stress and, conversely, positive emotion affect how we feel every moment of every day. An exploration of these concepts is necessary to develop a working understanding of the physiology underlying stress and the damage we are doing to ourselves when we live our lives from a constant state of stress. In addition, if we understand the damage caused by everyday stress, we can more easily assess the potential impact of creating the opposite circumstances in our daily lives.

Included in this chapter are specifics of the stress process. When we have a deep understanding of the vast damage we are doing to ourselves by the stresses to which we continually expose ourselves, we are more motivated to change. Our look at the stress process includes a brief examination of the stress hormone cortisol and some of its damaging effects. When we realize the destructive effects of cortisol on our health and on the way we think and act, we are much more able to grasp the potential effects of oxytocin. Oxytocin, which has been referred to as the calm and connection hormone,[1] is produced by, among other things, positive trusting and loving emotions. The potential effects of oxytocin will be discussed in Chapter Six.

Also included in this chapter is a brief review of the overall negative effects of stress on our health, specifically on our immune system, cognition—or how we process and reason—and memory. Also of import is the way the developing brain processes stress, as demonstrated by research examining the brains of adolescents and young adults. The plasticity of the brain is of fundamental concern in our transformative process, and at the end of the chapter, we begin to comprehend how repeated patterns of emotion influence our cognitive ability and, more importantly, imprint our brain for further development.

As much of this chapter briefly reviews current research in selected areas of stress, a good deal of the original terminology is kept intact. However, I have done my best to take scientific concepts and make them more comprehensible to underscore how these concepts have a profound impact on the way we live. I encourage you to take some time to digest and understand the significance of the concepts presented. When we understand the damage we are doing to ourselves every day by the choices we make, we can more easily understand how we can live from a more internally coherent and productive state. This state requires turning inward and consistently and intentionally redirecting our emotional attention to grateful, loving, and compassionate states, or intentionally cultivating a higher level of internal experience.

The outer paths of a labyrinth prepare one for the journey ahead. On the outskirts of our journey, as represented in Chapter Two, we defined and differentiated the concepts of stress, anxiety, and associated terms. Understanding these distinctions is of primary importance in the further examination of the process and consequences of stress and anxiety, and this understanding lays the groundwork necessary to grasp the importance of paying attention to our emotionally reactive patterns and the choices of where we keep our emotional attention every moment of every day.

Now we turn to the stress response. The stress response is a physiological and biochemical reality. In other words, when we feel stress, we undergo very real and consuming physical and chemical reactions in our bodies and brains. These responses may literally prevent us from thinking clearly, from acting in appropriate and loving ways, and from accessing and operating from the guidance of our internal selves. The static of stress, anxiety, and emotional unease may block the path to our own internal wisdom, calm, and productivity. The static of stress, anxiety, and emotional unease only lead to chaotic internal experience, and as you will discover throughout this book, our repeated internal experience becomes our way of being in the world.

Stress and anxiety perpetuate themselves. As we consistently and routinely expose ourselves to the physiology, biochemistry, and energetics of stress and anxiety, significant physical adaptations occur in our bodies and brains that continue and worsen the stress cycle. We literally become more biologically capable of experiencing increased stress and begin to suffer increasing resultant negative effects from that stress. As will be demonstrated in this chapter, these negative effects can have significant implications for our physical and mental health, our relationships, and our lives. The perpetuating cycle of stress and anxiety and resultant adaptations are important considerations on our journey. Our labyrinth is now gaining meaning.

The General Impact of Stress

The stress and anxiety responses are very real, scientifically measurable, physiological responses to a perceived stressor. That is, when we perceive anything to be a threat, be it internal or external, our bodies react in physically measurable and predictable ways. Physical, emotional, and behavioral responses to stress and anxiety are intimately related. The more intense the emotional response, the stronger the physical response, and the perception of the stressor's severity determines the emotional response.[2] According to Joseph LeDoux, "emotion can be defined as the process by which the brain determines or computes the value of a stimulus."[3]

Now, relate the overall stress response a person may feel to what we have learned about how anxiety is stored in our brains. When we perceive anything to be even remotely a threat, be it paying a bill, arguing with a partner, or taking a test, our brain looks for subconscious stored information, which may or may not be appropriate for the circumstance, and releases an emotional reaction. That reaction causes a flood of stress biochemicals throughout our bodies and sets off a cascade of brain synapse patterns that tells our bodies we need to react. Again, the stress response we are experiencing may be in much greater magnitude than is appropriate for the situation. Additionally, the stress response a person experiences can be chronic or acute. That is, "less dramatic, chronic, real-life situations evoke clear stress-related physiological responses as well as dramatic life events."[4] Whether it stems from seemingly insignificant but unrelenting stresses or a major life event, the stress response invokes a domino effect of physical reactions throughout our bodies and brains.

Two major physiological control systems work together and are activated by the stress response: the autonomic nervous system (ANS) and the endocrine system.[5] *Autonomic* basically means that these responses are automatic and not under conscious control. Feeling stressed stimulates automatic physical reactions throughout our body. The ANS controls, among other things, cardiovascular responses like heart rate, blood pressure, and something called heart rate variability. It also controls, with help of the endocrine system, various processes of targeted organs. Basically, the sympathetic division of the ANS stimulates body processes to speed up, and the parasympathetic slows things down.

The endocrine system is responsible for secreting hormones throughout the body. A hormone is a chemical substance that regulates specific bodily functions. We usually think of hormones as sex-related substances, but that is only one branch of hormones. As will be discussed in more depth in Chapter Four, we also have biochemicals called neurohormones, neuropeptides, and neurotransmitters that are intimately involved in emotion and the stress response. For now, understanding that when we are stressed we have an enormous release of biochemicals throughout our body is sufficient.

These two systems work in concert and trigger a series of profound physiological reactions in our bodies, including a whole host of cardiovascular and biochemical responses. Responses travel through nerves, with the help of biochemicals in activating cells and organs, and also as chemical messengers throughout the bloodstream. Under the control of the sympathetic division of the ANS, as well as key hormones released by the endocrine system, nearly every organ, sweat gland, blood vessel, and muscle—including the heart and brain—are profoundly affected.[6]

The Importance of Cortisol

Much will be said in this book about two specific hormones, cortisol and oxytocin, and their association with either stress or positive loving emotions. The importance of oxytocin will be addressed as we examine cultivating positive loving emotions. Cortisol, on the other hand, is usually considered the primary stress hormone. Although other hormones are associated with stress, like adrenalin (epinephrine) and norepinephrine, cortisol is more often studied because of the belief that it is the most damaging.

Cortisol has been associated with increased levels of blood sugar,[7] storage of body fat,[8] and increased aging.[9, 10] Cortisol has also been linked to other injurious effects throughout the body. Some of the more pertinent effects of cortisol in regard to our examination of emotion and transformation will be discussed shortly. First, let's examine a simplified representation of how cortisol is released.

According to Joseph LeDoux, when we perceive stress, the amygdala sends messages to the hypothalamus, which in turn sends messages to the pituitary gland to secrete a hormone called adrenocorticotropic hormone (ACTH). This hormone travels through the bloodstream to the adrenal cortex (Figure 3.1), which is part of the adrenal gland and sits on top of the kidney. The adrenal cortex is stimulated and, in turn, releases stress hormones.[11] Remember, the amygdala is the primary organ in our brain that stores anxiety and is hyperreactive to any perceived threat.

A primary class of stress hormones released through the adrenal cortex is called glucocorticoids; the primary glucocorticoid is cortisol. Cortisol raises blood sugar and mobilizes fatty acids. These responses are designed to mobilize energy sources to fight or flee. Unfortunately, in our current culture we don't usually need the extent of these resources to combat the stress to which we are exposed, and this response becomes more harmful than helpful.

If the fatty acids are utilized, they pose little risk, but if they remain in the blood system, they may contribute to a heart attack or the development of heart disease. These fatty acids also may be redistributed closer to where they are likely to be used, namely near the liver or as abdominal fat.[12] Blood sugar levels above normal can lead to the development and onset of diabetes.

The body is extremely adaptable and adjusts to what we continually give it. Unfortunately, when the body remains stressed, it adapts by creating the capability to produce even more cortisol. Hormone synthesis is a complicated process, but let's consider a basic explanation. Hormones and other biochemicals bind to specific receptor sites on the surface of target cells. Receptors recognize only one type of biochemical, in this case a specific hormone; they are usually found on the surface membrane of the target cell and cause the release of a second messenger inside the cell. One characteristic that determines whether a cell responds to a particular hormone—such as adrenocorticotropic hormone (ACTH),

ENDOCRINE SYSTEM

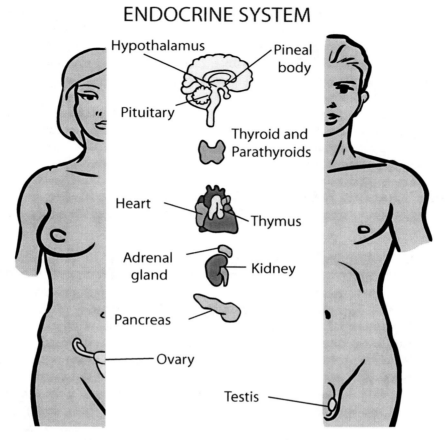

FIGURE 3.1 Anatomy of the adrenal cortex and its relation to the brain.

which controls the production of cortisol—is the amount of receptors manufactured by that cell and inserted into the membrane. Thus, only the cells that produce the appropriate receptors respond to specific hormones.

These hormone receptors can increase or decrease in number in response to need, and this process is usually referred to as *up-regulation* or *down-regulation*. The pituitary, in response to a perceived stressor, releases ACTH. A main characteristic of most hormonal systems, in addition to manufacturing hormones, is that they also detect and evaluate a hormone's effects. Secretion is up-regulated as an appropriate response to the amount of receptor sites being created. Large amounts of ACTH promote a proliferation and growth of adrenal cortical cells, increasing the capacity to produce even more stress hormones, including cortisol.[13]

Ongoing stress results in chronically elevated levels of ACTH, more receptor sites, and resultant elevated levels of cortisol and other stress hormones. In other words, the more we experience stress and anxiety, the more biologically capable we are to keep perpetuating and increasing those states. Additionally, more receptor sites on the cells may actually stimulate the body to create more cortisol and regard this elevated level as the new homeostasis. In essence, our cells may become addicted to the negative biochemical reactions taking place, produce more receptor sites for those specific hormones, and create a physiological and psychological need to fill those sites.

In effect, we become addicted to the perpetual cortisol baths we expose ourselves to. This may become a familiar place, but not a healthy one. Conversely, if these negative biochemical reactions can be replaced with positive biochemical reactions, such as those involving oxytocin, receptor sites with an affinity for oxytocin and like hormones are created and a new, lower level of stress baseline is established. Thus, the body strives to keep that much healthier balance as the preferred homeostasis. In addition, as will be shared in more depth later, it appears that higher levels of oxytocin actually reduce the stress response by blocking the effects of cortisol.

Stress in Research: Health Implications

Research has clearly shown a link between mental and emotional attitudes, stress and physiological health. For example, according to a Mayo Clinic study of individuals with heart disease, psychological stress was the strongest predictor of future cardiac events, as measured by cardiac arrest and cardiac death.[14] Other research on the results of three 10-year studies found that emotional stress was more predictive of death from cancer and cardiovascular disease than was smoking. Additionally, the results of those studies indicated that people who were unable to effectively manage their stress had a 40 percent higher death rate than those who felt they effectively managed stress.[15] Furthermore, high levels of stress hormones can increase the work of the heart. As high levels of stress hormones signal a fight or flight reaction, the body's metabolism is diverted away from the type of tissue repair needed to cure heart disease.[16]

Clearly, emotional stress has been linked to long-term detrimental health effects and reduced quality of life. In addition to the physiological ramifications of stress, there is a multitude of negative psycho-physiological effects. In other words, emotional stress damages both our physical and psychological health. These negative effects may contribute to the development of depression and can severely inhibit cognitive functioning, or the ability to think and reason clearly.[17]

According to the National Institute of Mental Health (NIMH), stress and depression are important risk factors for heart disease, along with high blood cholesterol and high blood pressure. Additionally, it appears that while chronically elevated levels of stress may cause depression, depression also contributes to chronically elevated levels of stress hormones, and both may have an impact on cognition. Effective therapies for depression and chronic stress may lie in breaking this harmful, self-perpetuating pattern and creating an intentional, positive emotional shift designed to reduce circulating stress hormones and increase hormones associated with calm and connection. If stress causes and perpetuates a negative internal experience, intentionally cultivating a higher internal experience shows great promise to reduce and replace these negative effects.

Stress and the Immune System

Stress-related psychological factors also have a great effect on the immune system. Under stressful conditions a continual release of cortisol has been shown to suppress the body's immunological responses. Additionally, it has been found that the competence of the immune system is decreased during depression, and such a compromise increases susceptibility to infectious diseases, cancer, and autoimmune disorders.[18]

Basically, when we are stressed or depressed, our immune system does not function optimally and we are much more likely to get sick—or worse. Long-term stress has an enormous impact on the immune system. I use the example of how many times students push and push throughout the quarter and then get sick during finals week or over quarter break. I have had significant experience with this concept. Some time ago, after a period of several years where I experienced considerable stress, my immune system was so depleted that I spent a period of several months very ill, seemingly catching any virus in my vicinity.

Fortunately, there is hope. Some research has examined the difference in secretory IgA (S-IgA) levels in self-induced and externally induced states of anger, or conversely, care and compassion. S-IgA is an immune system antibody important in the defense of specific bacteria and viruses. The more S-IgA you have, the more your immune system is vibrant and able to fight off infections. In this research, self-induced anger produced a significant increase in total mood disturbance and heart rate, but not S-IgA. Self-induced or intentionally activated care and compassion produced a significant decrease in total mood disturbance and a significant increase in S-IgA.[19]

Two significant points need to be addressed regarding this research. The first point is the significant increase in the immune system antibody S-IgA. In our lives we are constantly exposed to bacteria and viruses, and an increase in S-IgA helps the body's defense against these pathogens. Secondly, and more importantly, the emotional states that produced the significant increases in S-IgA were self-induced. What is key about this point is that the higher emotion and refocusing techniques, or HEART, presented in this book rest on making an intentional emotional shift to a positive and loving state. This research demonstrates that looking inward to find emotional states of care, compassion, and positive loving emotions can significantly change our physiology and our life.

Cognition

What is cognition? *Webster's Concise Medical Dictionary* defines cognition as "a generic term embracing the quality of knowing, which includes perceiving, recognizing, conceiving, judging, sensing, reasoning, and imagining."[20] The *Oxford Dictionary* defines cognition as "knowing, perceiving, or conceiving as an act or faculty."[21] According to the NIMH, cognition is a term that encompasses perception, attention, learning, memory, thought, and communication.[22] The general consensus is that cognition is a mental process of acquiring knowledge through reasoning or perception.

Given the consensus that cognition is fundamentally a mental process, what is the possible relationship between cognition, stress, and anxiety? Can a person's cognitive processes or ability at any given time be reduced or enhanced due to his or her physiological response to perceived stress? If an important aspect of cognition is perception, could cognition conversely affect a person's stress or anxiety level by his or her perception of that stress?

Stress, anxiety, and cognition are intrinsically related. It is impossible to effectively examine cognitive performance without considering the psycho-physiological impact of stress and anxiety. Additionally, it is essential, when examining stress and anxiety to include the role of perception, both as a precursor to stress and anxiety and a result of the stress and anxiety response. In other words, our perception of the severity of the stress determines our reaction, yet our reactive patterns also determine our perception of stress—and both have an impact on cognition.

In an effort to gain a deeper understanding of the impact of anxiety on cognitive performance, some research has examined interhemispheric processing in subjects differing in self-reported worry, under perceived high and low stress conditions. Anxiety is often defined as worry or apprehension, and in this case the subjects reported how much anxiety they felt under different levels of stressful conditions.

The brain is divided into two sides, or hemispheres. Across hemispheric advantage, or AHA, is the coordination of information between these two brain regions. AHA has been shown to enhance cognitive processing, or higher level thinking. In this research, the individuals identified as worriers showed significantly reduced efficiency of AHA, indicating that one source of impaired cognition associated with anxiety is the coordination of information between brain regions. Additionally, AHA was exaggerated under high stress conditions, indicating that interhemispheric processing becomes especially important under a higher stress load.[23]

The results of this study indicated high levels of worry-impaired cognition, and higher levels of worry impaired cognition even more. In short, anxiety and worry reduce our capabilities to think and reason. If we do not address the physiological implications of anxiety and the resultant effects of anxiety on cognition, we are not truly committed to performing our best. Furthermore, the physical effects of anxiety and negative emotional states linger.

Cognition and Emotion

In his paper on "Cognition, Emotion, and Other Inescapable Dimensions of Human Experience," Jorge Frascara argues that human cognitive performance is context dependent. In other words, human cognitive processes vary from situation to situation, and fear, anxiety, and stress impair performance in a usually proficient task. Additionally, Frascara argues that the emotional context of a situation changes the abstract concept of logical thinking.

He also suggests that an increase in arousal narrowly focuses the subject's attention. If this attention is appropriately based, then efficiency may occur. However, if this narrowing misses cues for appropriate choice, performance deteriorates. Furthermore, Frascara contends that training in cognitive tasks, without taking into account training in emotional control, does little to assure the proper functioning of that task under stressful conditions. Finally, he asserts that emotional states affect people's skills and cognitive performance and people in good moods have higher expectations about their ability to achieve positive outcomes.[24]

These considerations have important implications for cognitive learning tasks regarding optimal performance, thinking, and reasoning clearly. In addition to Frascara's assertions about missing important cues, the theory of "inattentional blindness" holds that we may literally miss visually perceiving items that don't receive focused attention. In other words, we perceive and remember only those objects and details that receive focused attention.[25]

If we literally see only what we pay attention to—and under stressful conditions that attention may be focused on past failure, expectations of current failure, or negative emotional states—we may literally miss seeing important avenues for success. Additionally, specific methods to increase performance may not be as effective as intended without also taking into account the context-specific emotional and mood environment surrounding the required tasks. Techniques to increase emotional resilience and reduce the stress and anxiety response may be much more effective in creating the emotional environment necessary for optimal cognitive functioning instead of just cognitive, academic, or performance strategies alone.

What all this boils down to is that our brains function better and we reason and process more efficiently when we are less anxious. We can more clearly see optimistic solutions when we are in a positive emotional state, and we are much more productive. When we choose to redirect our feeling state inward to create calm, centered, and connected emotional states, or a higher internal experience, we function better, think more clearly, and perform at our best.

Memory

It is a common experience that stressful events influence cognitive performance. Physiologically, a significant influencing factor seems to be a function of cortical inhibition—that is, the inhibition of the neocortex, or "thinking" part of the brain. This inhibition seems to stem from glucocorticoid and catecholamine hormones secreted by the adrenal cortex during and after a stressful event. In other words, when we are stressed, our adrenal glands release stress hormones into the blood, which carries them to the brain and influence its functioning.

Research has turned up conflicting findings about memory and stress. Some studies have shown memory retrieval, or the ability to remember stored information, is inhibited during stress, and other research has shown enhanced memory consolidation, or strengthening emotional memory storage.

There are fundamental differences in memory consolidation and memory retrieval, and understanding these differences is important when examining anxiety. As we have noted, anxiety is most often defined as the apprehension of a fearful or stressful event, usually involving dread or perceived danger. The experience of this apprehension is believed to be caused by significantly emotional memories stored in the limbic portion, specifically the amygdala, of the brain. Thus, memory consolidation—specifically, the storage of emotional memory—is the foundation of this process. Why then, when we experience anxiety, do we often experience a lapse in memory, such as when we are taking an important exam?

Cognitive memory retrieval, or needing to recall important stored cognitive information, is a very different physiological process than emotional memory storage or consolidation.

Making a distinction between these two forms of memory is paramount in understanding anxiety. Though their functions are profoundly different, they can occur simultaneously, and one form (consolidation) can exacerbate the other (impaired retrieval). Additionally, understanding this process is fundamentally important in comprehending how chronic or acute anxiety contributes to reduced cognition through impaired memory retrieval and how it further exacerbates negative emotional memory storage.

Recent research reviewed the current findings regarding the acute effects of glucocorticoids on the storage of emotional memory and information retrieval. These findings come from the Center for the Neurobiology of Learning and Memory at the University of California, Irvine. The evidence suggests that the consequences of glucocorticoids on cognition depends largely on the memory phases being investigated, more specifically, memory consolidation or memory retrieval.

The findings indicate that memory consolidation is enhanced by glucocorticoid-sensitive pathways similar to that of catecholamines—that is, by activation of the amygdala and storage of emotional memory. However, memory retrieval is impaired, reducing retention performance, while glucocorticoids are still high. Additionally, this research shows that the acute effects of glucocorticoids may also partly explain the detrimental long-term effects of anxiety on cognitive performance in the area of contextual or declarative information and in patients with schizophrenia or depression.[26]

It is important to note that in cognition memory retrieval and memory consolidation occur simultaneously. Thus, a single corticoid rush can enhance emotional memory consolidation of a specific upsetting event, while simultaneously impairing retrieval of previously stored information. For example, the physiological effects of anxiety may cause memory retrieval to be temporarily disrupted during an important exam; however, strong and vivid memories of this experience may endure a lifetime. In other words, we can't remember information we know, but our bodies and subconscious minds will never forget that emotional experience!

It is also plausible that the disruption of information retrieval during stressful conditions may actually facilitate the storage of the emotional memory during such arousing experiences.[27] In other words, if we're doing something important and we're so stressed we draw a blank, we'll never forget the emotional experience of not being able to recall crucial information at that point! The detrimental effects of glucocorticoids produced from stressful events are of primary importance in examining anxiety. At this point in our evolution, we no longer need to run away from a tiger, but we do need to think during a test or perform at our cognitive best.

Furthermore, the effects of glucocorticoids on memory retrieval are only one aspect of their injurious effects. High levels of circulating cortisol also can have profound effects on brain biochemistry and actually perpetuate the anxiety cycle. As we learned in Chapter Two, anxiety is stored in the limbic/amygdala area of the brain and becomes an automatic subconscious response the next time we are exposed to that or a similar stressor. As this research shows, memory consolidation, or the storage of emotional memory, is a response to acute or chronic stress.

What this research shows is that the process of anxiety is greatly exaggerated under stressful conditions. Again, once the emotional memory is stored, the anxiety response becomes automatic and begins a whole host of physiological, systemwide responses. If we don't have the tools to redirect our emotional attention, we may get caught up in a perpetuating cycle of stress and anxiety that inhibits our performance and our lives.

Brain Adaptations and the Perpetuating Cycle of Stress

It has been well established that glucocorticoids in general and cortisol in particular are important contributors to the stress response and may lead to greater anxiety, reduced memory and cognition, depression, and many other negative physiological effects. The body has incredible adaptation abilities and in many situations will modify its physiology in response to the increasing demands placed upon it. Prolonged periods of stress and anxiety can be problematic as the body goes through physiological and biochemical adaptations within the brain itself that serve to facilitate more cortisol. A basic understanding of this process helps underscore the importance of reducing the influx of negative emotions.

According to Joe Dispenza, "nerve cells that fire together wire together."[28] In other words, if we do something over and over again, the brain synapse patterns that are firing from that behavior begin to establish a neural network and "carve a track in the brain." If we do something long enough, this neural network gets stronger and stronger and begins to become hardwired in the brain. Our habits become who we are. If we are constantly focused on stress and anxiety, this becomes our way of being in the world. What may seem like an innocent need to retell our "stories" to gain sympathy or be "the drama queen" is actually a message to our brain to make sure we really begin to play that role.

In addition to strengthening negative brain reaction patterns, chronic stress or negative thought patterns actually perpetuate the anxiety cycle. Again, according to Dispenza, chronic stress causes the glucocorticoids released in our system to influence the production of noradrenalin, a hormone related to adrenalin. Noradrenalin communicates with the amygdala, the emotional center of the brain, which releases more CRH, or corticotropic releasing hormone, which starts the process explained in Chapter Two all over again.

The hippocampus is supposed to regulate the amount of glucocorticoids released by the action of its steroid receptors in an attempt to match the amount of stress hormones to the stress stimulus, but this is not always the case. Under optimal conditions, the hippocampus detects the amount of glucocorticoids in its receptor sites and sends messages to the hypothalamus and pituitary to slow down production. However, when the amygdala is overactivated by chronic or unresolved stress, or stress caused by constantly catastrophizing, the hippocampus begins to falter in its ability to temper the release of stress hormones.[29] Thus, the destructive, circular, and perpetuating pattern of stress continues.

Genetic Predisposition?

Admittedly, there are genetic predispositions observed in some who succumb to stress related conditions that are different from those who do not. Higher trait anxious individuals may have a genetic predisposition to be that way. A study of 1,037 people who were followed for many years through multiple episodes of stress uncovered a correlation between the long and the short forms of SERT and the likelihood of developing depression. SERT is a 5-HTT serotonin transporter gene that had been identified in earlier studies as a contributing factor, and possible identifier, of those who would succumb to depression or anxiety disorders after periods of chronic stress. The subjects in this study who had the short form of SERT and who reported a five-year history of three or four life stressors were more likely to develop depression or anxiety disorders than those who had the long form of this gene.[30]

While considering the previous study, on the surface a genetic predisposition to trait anxiety and depression seems to dictate a negative outcome. However, this fatalistic attitude may be unwarranted due to two important considerations. First, a significant amount of ongoing stress may be required to activate this gene. Again, the stress response is the physiological reaction to a perceived stressor. While many times we cannot change a life stressor, it is possible with intervention to change our perception of that stressor and thus reduce the physiological reaction to that stressor. Additionally, chronic low levels of stress have also been linked to depression. Interventions specifically directed at reducing the body's cortisol production during these times of stress may have an impact on restructuring the body's stress response and helping to reduce depressive episodes.[31]

A second, exceptionally important consideration in the examination of this genetic predisposition lies in its reactivity. It is hypothesized that the reason this short form of SERT contributes to anxiety and depression is that it is hyperreactive to the stress response and is activated by chronic, low-grade "cortisol baths."[32] Research on genetic predisposition is in its initial stages. Identification of this gene and its link to anxiety and depression have just recently been discovered.

What is fundamentally important in this reactivity hypothesis is that it is believed that this gene may also be hyperreactive to intervention techniques. National Institute of Mental Health (NIMH) researchers theorize that this genetic predisposition to depression and anxiety may also predispose a person to significant improvement through intervention.[33] This possible improvement through appropriate intervention techniques aimed at reducing cortisol is a new and potentially enlightening direction for future research. In other words, learning to redirect our emotional attention from states of anxiety and fear by intentionally cultivating higher emotional states, including those caused by turning inward and sincerely feeling care, compassion, and positive loving emotions, may help to control this genetic predisposition.

This research underscores the important work of Bruce Lipton, who challenges the long-held assumption that genes alone control our biology. His work documents the fact that genes are often activated, or not, by what is going on biochemically and energetically in our bodies as a result to the thoughts and feelings we display every day.[34] SERT the 5-HTT serotonin transporter gene is evidence of this fact. It appears this gene can be activated by low-grade constant cortisol baths, which can be created by focusing our emotional attention on all the things that are wrong or could go wrong.

Special Considerations for Infants, Adolescents, Teens, and Young Adults

This examination of the physiology and psychophysiology of stress and anxiety so far has been on what we know from adult populations and infer as the physiological reality for adolescents and children. However, some aspects of the stress response may differ with reduced chronological age. Of special consideration when examining stress and anxiety in children, adolescents, and young adults is the crucial fact that their brains are still developing.

In a discussion of stress and the developing brain, NIMH researchers theorize that early influences (i.e., negative experiences and chronic stressors) may affect a young child's developing brain. Of specific concern is the cortisol released over a long time span on the developing brain. Additionally, these researchers suggest that long-term effects of excess cortisol may cause shrinking of the hippocampus, a brain structure required for the formation of certain types of memory.[35]

After examining the neurobiological factors that may contribute to the exaggeration of the stress response in adolescence, research has shown that adolescence is a particularly vulnerable period for stress-induced prefrontal cortical functioning; even mild uncontrollable stress impairs the cognitive functioning of the prefrontal cortex in an adolescent.[36] The prefrontal cortex is a brain region critical for insight, judgment, and the inhibition of inappropriate behaviors.

In addition to damage to the developing brain caused by excess cortisol, there is evidence that the anatomy of the developing brain, in comparison to the adult brain, may lend itself to higher degrees of anxiety and reactivity. The NIMH, in a brief overview of research examining brain development and teens, reports that the use of magnetic resonance imaging (MRI) revealed previously unrecognized patterns of brain development in the teenage years, and these differences in developmental stages may play a crucial role in the relationship of anxiety and cognition. The NIMH report, *The Teenage Brain: A Work in Progress,* asserts that by following the same brains from childhood through adolescence and into young adulthood, we now have a much deeper understanding of the changing nature of the brain.[37] These MRI studies have employed the technique of scanning a child's brain every two years to reveal typical biological changes that take place over time in the human brain.

Evidence shows that the increased myelination and maturation of the frontal lobe doesn't occur until young adulthood; this area of the brain relates to cognitive processing and other executive functions. UCLA researchers found that the frontal lobe of the brain showed the largest differences between teens (12 to 16 years old) and young adults (23 to 30 years old) and hypothesized that the increase in myelination in the adult frontal cortex likely relates to the maturation of cognitive processing. Myelination speeds transmission of information through the neuron.

Additionally, young teens, while undergoing an emotional task, were found to activate the amygdala more than the frontal lobe.[38] The amygdala promotes fear and emotional arousal and is associated with anxiety and gut reactions, while the frontal cortex mediates this response, leading to more reasoned perceptions. Thus, these studies indicate a more emotionally driven, less-reasoned response behavior pattern in adolescence through young adulthood.

This research regarding teen and adolescent brain development underscores the importance of programs to reduce the stress response in developing brains. We know from evidence stemming from adult research that stress and anxiety can have deleterious effects on cognition, memory, and overall health. It appears that the young adult, teen, and adolescent brain may be even more prone to those harmful effects due to increased activation of the amygdala and reduced capacity of the frontal cortex. Additionally, excess cortisol on the developing brain of a child may have profound implications for the child throughout his or her life if interventions to change that stress response are not implemented.

Direct research on the physiology of stress in children and adolescents is not always possible. Aside from the assumptions we make regarding these populations from research on adults, we also theorize based on animal research. Research on animals has shown that stress-induced young rats were shown to have a more profound and excessive stress response in subsequent tests than controls. This excessive response appeared to last into adulthood; however, exposure to an enriched setting seems to reverse this trend.[39] This appears to suggest that negative and stressful environments perpetuate and exacerbate the stress response, while positive environments reduce this same response.

From the research on children, adolescents, and young adults, it is apparent that environments infused with positive emotional environments are much more optimal than those infused with stress and anxiety. From the research on the plasticity of the brain, it appears that even if the circumstances during development have not been optimal, there is still hope for change. Most of this research points to the fact that the conditions for change, or transformation, need to come from within. In other words, even when external circumstances improve, if negative thought and emotional patterns remain, there is little hope for lasting improvement.

Continuing on the Path

Returning to our metaphor of the labyrinth, this chapter gives meaning and depth to our journey to the center by exploring the body's overall stress response. In other words, when the brain either consciously or subconsciously perceives a threat, we experience a physical reaction that involves the whole body.

It is important to remember that the anxiety response can be triggered by internal stimuli, like the pressure we put on ourselves, or by our perceptions of external circumstances. Remember, too, that we may not be aware of what is setting off that reaction even as we experience it in our bodies.

What we feel is the stress response—a whole body response activated in milliseconds through the integration of our nervous and endocrine systems, and we know it because we feel it. Where we keep our attention profoundly affects the anxiety and stress responses in our bodies, and routine attention to anything creates stronger neural networks in our brains that make it easier to remain in those states.

In Chapter Four we will demonstrate how these responses deeply affect how we feel at any given moment and how we have the power of choice. Chapter Five begins to explore the power of emotion. All of the information up to that point becomes synthesized when we look at the process of emotion and the power of looking inward to consciously create positive and higher emotions.

One of the most impressive discoveries in neuroscience over the last decade is that the parts of the brain involved in anxiety, fear, and emotion change in response to experience.[40] This is evidence of the neuroplasticity of the brain. Additionally, recent research indicates that those same parts of the brain are associated with higher emotional states such as love, gratitude, and trust. The power for transformation comes from realizing we have the capability of creating our own internal experiences, and these experiences profoundly affect our quality of life. The power lies within.

REFERENCES

1. Uvnas Moberg, K., *The Oxytocin Factor: Tapping the Hormone of Love, Calm, and Healing* (Cambridge, MA: Perseus, 2003).

2. Cowley, G., "Our Bodies, Our Fears," in special edition on Anxiety and Our Brain, *Newsweek,* February 24, 2003, 44–49.

3. LeDoux, J., *The Synaptic Self: How Our Brains Become Who We Are* (New York: Viking, 2002).

4. Donatelle, R. J., *Health: The Basics,* 4th ed. (Boston: Allyn and Bacon, 2001).

5. Rosenzweig, M., A. L. Leiman, and S. M. Breedlove, *Biological Psychology: An Introduction to Behavioral, Cognitive, and Clinical Neuroscience,* 2nd ed. (Sunderland, MA: Sinauer Associates, 1999).

6. Ibid.

7. DeFeo, P., "Contribution of Cortisol to Glucose Counterregulation in Humans," *American Journal of Physiology 257* (1989): E35–E42.

8. Marin, P., et al., "Cortisol Secretion in Relation to Body Fat Distribution in Obese Premenopausal Women," *Metabolism 41* (1992): 882–886.

9. Namiki, M., "Aged People and Stress," *Japanese Journal of Geriatrics 31:2* (1994): 85–95.

10. Kerr, D. S., et al., "Chronic Stress-Induced Acceleration of Electrophysiologic and Morphometric Biomarkers of Hippocampal Aging," *Journal of Neuroscience 11:5* (1991): 1316–1324.

11. LeDoux, J., *The Emotional Brain: The Mysterious Underpinnings of Emotional Life* (New York: Simon and Schuster, 1996).

12. Girdano, D. A., D. E. Dusek, and G. S. J. Everly, *Controlling Stress and Tension* (San Francisco: Pearson/Benjamin Cummings, 2005).

13. Rosenzweig, Leiman, and Breedlove, *Biological Psychology.*

14. Allison, T. G., et al., "Medical and Economic Costs of Psychologic Distress in Patients with Coronary Artery Disease," *Mayo Clinic Proceedings 70:8* (1995): 734–742.

15. Eysenck, H. J., "Personality, Stress and Cancer: Prediction and Prophylaxis," *British Journal of Medical Psychology 61* (Pt 1) (1988): 57–75.

16. Nemeroff, C. B., D. L. Musselman, and D. L. Evans, "Depression and Cardiac Disease," *Depression and Anxiety, 8* (suppl 1) (1998): 71–79.

17. Ibid.

18. Stein, M., and A. H. Miller, "Depression, the Immune System, and Health and Illness: Findings in Search of Meaning," *Archives of General Psychiatry 48* (1991): 171–177.

19. Rein, G., M. Atkinson, and R. McCraty, "The Physiological and Psychological Effects of Compassion and Anger," *Journal of Advancement in Medicine 8:2* (1995): 87–105.

20. Hensyl, W.R., ed. *Webster's New World/Stedman's Concise Medical Dictionary* (New York: Simon and Schuster, 1987).

21. Abate, F. R., ed. *The Oxford Dictionary and Thesaurus.* (New York: Oxford University Press, 1997).

22. National Institute of Mental Health (NIMH), *Cognitive Research at the National Institute of Mental Health* (Bethesda, MD: Author, 2000).

23. Compton, R. J., and D. A. Mintzer, "Effects of Worry and Evaluation Stress on Interhemispheric Interaction," *Neuropsychology 15:4* (2001): 427–433.

24. Frascara, J., "Cognition, Emotion, and Other Inescapable Dimensions of Human Experience," *Visible Language 33:1* (1999): 74–89.

25. Simons, D. J., and C. F. Chabris, "Gorillas in Our Midst: Sustained Inattentional Blindness for Dynamic Events," *Perception 28* (1999): 1059–1074.

26. Roozendaal, B., "Stress and Memory: Opposing Effects of Glucocorticoids on Memory Consolidation and Memory Retrieval," *Neurobiology of Learning and Memory 78* (2002): 578–595.

27. Ibid.

28. Arntz, W., B. Chasse, and M. Vicente, *What the Bleep Do We Know!?* (Deerfield Beach, FL: Health Communications, 2003), 171.

29. LeDoux, *Emotional Brain.*

30. NIMH, *Cognitive Research.*

31. NIMH, *National Advisory Mental Health Council (Minutes from the 204th Meeting)* (Bethesda, MD: Author, 2003).

32. NIMH, *Cognitive Research.*

33. Ibid.

34. Lipton, B. *The Biology of Belief: Unleashing the Power of Consciousness, Matter, and Miracles* (Santa Rosa, CA: Mountain of Love, 2005).

35. Sheline, Y. I., et al., "Depression Duration But Not Age Predicts Hippocampal Volume Loss in Medically Healthy Women with Recurrent Major Depression," *Journal of Neuroscience 19:12* (1999): 5034–5043.

36. Arnsten, A. F., and R. M. Shansky, "Adolescence: Vulnerable Period for Stress-Induced Prefrontal Cortical Function?" *Annals of the New York Academy of Sciences 1021* (2004): 143–147.

37. National Institute of Health, *Teenage Brain: A Work in Progress* (Bethesda, MD: Author, 2001).

38. Ibid.

39. Jones, T. A., et al., "Induction of Multiple Synapses by Experience in the Visual Cortex of Adult Rats," *Neurobiology of Learning and Memory 68:1* (1997): 13–20.

40. Girdano, Dusek, and Everly, *Controlling Stress.*

CHAPTER four

The "Feeling" States of Stress

Introduction

A critical concept—and a recurrent theme throughout this book—is that where we have our emotional attention, whether by choice or by circumstance, profoundly affects the way we feel at any given moment. Grasping the concept that how we physically feel is powerfully connected to where we have our emotional attention is the beginning step to transformation.

In Chapter Three we examined how our bodies and psyches strongly react in a physical sense to our thoughts and emotional reactions. These reactions can be from reactive patterns buried in our brains; they may or not be appropriate for the circumstance, but the feeling of unease, or worse, that we experience throughout our bodies and the physical implications of that feeling are very real.

The following exercise is designed to help you grasp this concept at a deeper level than you would experience from just reading about it. It is important to engage at a meaningful level with this exercise and write about personal experiences that carried a significant amount of feeling response.

The Feeling States of Emotion
EXERCISE AND REFLECTION #2

Write vividly about a time you felt particularly stressed. It does not have to be the most severe time of stress in your life, although it can be if that's what you choose to write about. It can be a smaller event that happened recently where you felt particularly stressed. The key is to choose a time where you experienced the emotional uneasiness of stress and describe the event in as much detail as possible. Write within the following guidelines:

1. Describe in as much detail as you can the specifics of the event.

_____

_____

_____

_____

_____

_____

_____

_____

_____

_____

_____

_____

_____

2. Describe how you generally felt psychologically and physically through this event or time period.

_____

_____

_____

_____

_____

_____

3. Describe any specific physical sensations you felt during this event or time period (e.g., headache, racing heart, pit in stomach).

_____

_____

_____

_____

_____

4. How do you physically feel right now, recalling the event? Do any of the physical symptoms resurface?

_____

_____

_____

STOP. Pause a minute to process and reflect.

Take a few deep breaths and try to clear your thought process. Now write about a time when you felt particularly happy, "in the zone," a time where you felt everything was flowing effortlessly. Again, this doesn't have to be the "high point" of your life, although it can be if you choose it to be. The time you write about should be one where you truly felt the sensations of happiness and coherence. Again, write within the following guidelines clearly and vividly.

1. Describe the event or time period in as much vivid detail as possible.

_____

_____

_____

_____

_____

_____

_____

_____

_____

_____

_____

_____

_____

_____

2. Describe how you generally felt psychologically and physically throughout this event or time period.

_____

_____

_____

_____

_____

_____

3. Describe any specific physical sensations you felt during this event or time period (focus in on the bodily sensations that accompanied this specific emotional state).

_____

_____

_____

_____

_____

4. How do you physically feel right now, recalling the event?

_____

_____

_____

STOP. Pause a minute to process and reflect.

Process/Reflect

Process and reflect in a way that is meaningful to you. You might find it helpful to process using the following protocol and addressing the following questions.

Read over what you have written. Brainstorm and write specific one- or two-word descriptions of how you felt during each time period or event, especially your physical reactions. Address the following questions:

1. How easy was it to think of something to write about and how enthusiastically did you begin writing (a) about the stressful event or time and (b) about the happy event or time?

2. If at all possible, retell the event to another person, complete with the general and specific psychological and physical reactions. How did you feel retelling the story?

3. What was your body language as you wrote about the stressful experience? What about the positive or happy experience? Your demeanor? What was the primary facial expression you were exhibiting as you wrote each story? How do you feel (not about the event itself, but physically and psychologically) right now? Are you experiencing some of the initial emotional reactions all over again?

Final Reflection

1. What was this whole experience like for you?

2. Were you more willing and able to focus on a negative event or time period than a positive event?

3. During the initial event, did you feel a psychological and physiological reaction to the event?

4. Did you experience the same feelings as you relived the experience? As you retold the experience?

5. If you retold the experience, how did you feel? If you listened to someone else retelling his or her experience, how did you relate to that retelling?

6. The theme of this exercise is to pay attention to our psychological and physiological demeanor as a response to where we choose to put our emotional attention. Can you relate to that theme? Did you find a lesson in this exercise?

Personal writing: Reflect, summarize, and process your response to the exercise and questions. What resonated with you most throughout this experience?

_____

_____

_____

_____

_____

_____

_____

_____

_____

_____

_____

_____

_____

_____

_____

_____

The "Feeling" States of Emotion

This is one of the most powerful exercises I do when I conduct workshops on stress management. I call it "The Feeling State of Stress." This exercise is significant because it illustrates, in a powerfully experiential way, the concept that our bodies and psyches are so profoundly affected by our positive or negative experiences that reliving, retelling, or focusing on those experiences often evokes those same reactions. The experience of this exercise underscores the fundamental concept that where we choose to place our emotional attention every minute of every day eventually becomes who we are.

The experience goes something like this. I ask participants to get out at least two sheets of blank paper. The intention behind the two blank sheets is that I want them to feel free to write whatever they need without a constrained space provided by me. Additionally, because the exercise is divided into two distinct halves, I want them to begin the second part on a separate sheet of paper to provide themselves the clearest energy field possible, uncontaminated by the first part of the activity.

On the first sheet I ask participants to write about a particularly stressful experience. The experience doesn't necessarily need to be the most stressful or difficult of their lives, although it can be if that's what they choose to write about. They need to be able to recall the experience clearly and connect with the feelings generated during that experience. Emphasizing the vivid detail is an important aspect, as I want to make sure participants are sincerely placing their emotional attention on retelling, in written form, their emotion-filled stories.

This recollection and examination process takes place in three stages. First, I ask participants to describe the stressful event or series of events in as much detail and with as much recall as they can. Second, I ask them to describe generally how they felt psychologically, emotionally, and physically during the stressful event. Finally, I direct them to pinpoint, if they can, their specific physical reactions to or during the event.

Generally, when I give the instructions to this part of the activity, participants are eager to begin. They write with energy and determination. They often write with anger, frustration, or a sense of defeat. I am fascinated by the body language and nonverbal communication being displayed as they write. Many participants clutch their pens so tightly their knuckles are turning white. Some angrily tap the floor with their feet, and others have their head in their hand as they write. I'm often curious about the amount of pressure their pens are exerting on the paper, as it looks excessive. The collective energy in the room begins to plummet.

Next, I ask if someone would be willing to share any or all of his or her story. I always emphasize that participants don't have to share if they are uncomfortable doing so, but note that it really helps the process of the activity if someone is willing to volunteer. Usually, someone does, after a short pause. Then, many more participants volunteer to share. It's almost as if they are trying to outdo each other in how challenging their stories are.

At this point the stories typically range from horrific life events to being stressed about more mundane things. In retelling their stories, participants begin to evoke emotional, psychological, and physical reactions similar to the initial event. I have had people cry, express anger, break their pencil, tighten their shoulders in knots, grit their teeth, and slump in their chair in despair. I usually have to cut the stories short because so many want to share.

As we begin to process the experience and as participants are sharing their stories, I am writing on the board descriptive words of their general experience. I quite often get words or phrases like overwhelmed, anxious, tired, frustrated, angry, and tense. "I felt like crying," participants say, or "I felt totally spent." Their descriptions of physical reactions often include comments like these:

My heart was racing.

I couldn't eat.

I got a headache.

I couldn't sleep.

I was anxious and tense all over.

My stomach felt like it was in a knot.

My neck hurt.

I was exhausted.

Unfortunately, the list goes on and on.

At this point I usually pause and ask a participant who has just shared how he or she is feeling at that moment of retelling the story. Occasionally, participants say they are relieved because they have worked through the difficult situation and are happy to be over it. But, when they understated that I am really asking how they are physically feeling at that moment, the vast percentage say they feel angry, stressed, or anxious all over again. Many feel as if they have reexperienced the event, physically and psychologically.

The energy in the room has plummeted. As I look around, I see many anxious, stressed, frustrated, and unhappy faces, complete with the body language to match. I ask the participants to just look around and observe the room and absorb the energy. Then I pause for a moment of silence to reflect.

Next, I ask participants to get out the other brand new piece of paper as to begin anew. On this sheet, I ask that they follow the same format, but this time they are to write about a time where they felt particularly happy, "in the zone," or as if everything was flowing effortlessly. I ask them to write about a time where they felt their life, situation, and bodies were operating coherently.

Again, the first step in this stage is to write about the time, situation, or event in as much vivid detail as possible. Step two is to describe in a general sense how they felt, and the third step is to specifically write how they felt in their bodies. Although the instructions are the same, the experience is very different.

What is immediately apparent is the participants' reluctance or inability to write. Some sit as if they can't think of anything to write. Others write a sentence or two and then stop as if nothing will flow, and a few remark that they truly can't allow themselves to write about anything good. Some even exhibit a nervous laugh.

After several minutes, most begin to write. The process of allowing themselves to focus vividly on a time when they really felt good comes slowly, but gradually the majority seems to shift and begins to focus. A few continue to struggle.

As the participants get more involved in their writing, their body language begins to shift. Some sit taller, some don't grip their pen so tightly, and some actually begin to smile and become quite engaged. The whole energy in the room seems to shift, but I keep quiet about what I am observing. The participants continue writing.

At the end of this process, I ask again if anyone is willing to share their story or any part of the writing activity. Typically, participants are much more reluctant during this phase of the activity. It's almost as if they are not culturally allowed to admit to times of feeling good. Some seem almost ready to volunteer but hesitant and embarrassed to acknowledge to the others in the group that they have had positive experiences. It's so much more comfortable to share their negative experiences.

Eventually someone volunteers, and if the story is an engaging one to which other participants can relate, the story seems to generate a collective shift in energy. Once one person has shared and the atmosphere in the room becomes lighter, there are many more volunteers. The people listening are usually quite engaged, and the storytelling becomes infectious. Participants are smiling, laughing, and truly absorbed in each other's stories.

Many of the words of the general description they experienced are like these:

I felt light.

I felt like everything was flowing.

I felt invincible.

I was happy

I felt calm, even transcendent.

Quite often participants retell their stories with a genuine smile, a complete shift in body language, and a visible transformation of attitude.

After several stories, or one or two very meaningful stories, the atmosphere of the room has undergone such a complete shift that participants begin to talk about how they are feeling. Many express disbelief about this shift in emotions. "I would never have believed this shift was possible if you had just told us about it," they say. "I came in with a horrible headache, but now I feel really happy."

Something important has happened through our experience, and it would never have been possible without the actual experience of genuinely engaging in the activity. The lessons learned through this activity exist on many different levels of awareness. The first and most obvious lesson is how events in our lives, whether they are happy or stressful, carry with them a profound and definite physical and psychological reaction. We feel the emotional experience in our bodies in a noticeable and definite way. This reaction underscores the central point of this book that stress and anxiety, and conversely happy times, carry with them a whole cascade of psychological and physiological reactions that invade our bodies, change our perceptions, and transform who we are at that moment, whether positive or negative.

A second lesson arises when I point out how enthusiastically the participants were willing to engage in writing about a stressful or unhappy time in their lives and almost unable to write about a time when they felt happy. I point out how they grabbed their pens and pencils tightly and began to write about the stressful event before I even finished giving directions. I also call attention to their reluctance, how they looked around, paused after one sentence, and in general seemed to feel discomfort as I asked them to share a happy or coherent time. The participants usually nod or laugh in agreement of that realization, as they are beginning to understand the depth of the lessons they have just experienced.

At this point I share what I observed in body language, feet tapping angrily, pencils breaking, general scowls, and the collective environment of the room as they were writing their stressful stories. A few will laugh out loud as they realize they were a prime example. Then, of course, I share the collective shift in verbal and nonverbal behavior and the apparent transformation of attitudes as they wrote about their positive events. This brings the experience to a much deeper level and to the third, all-important lesson of this activity.

I tell them, "I just intentionally manipulated your emotions."

They begin to look back half in disbelief and half in genuine recognition of the fact that they have just experienced an intense feeling of and shift in emotional behavior, complete with all the profound psychological and physiological changes they experienced. My query usually goes something like this: "What's changed? We're still in the same seats, with the same pieces of paper and pen or pencils as we were an hour ago. All I did was ask you to participate in an activity where you chose to focus your emotional attention on a specific event. By focusing your emotional attention on these events, many of you felt as if you relived that event at a psychological and physiological level, complete with mood, perception, and environmental shifts to match. That shift happened through a stressful recollection as well as a happy recollection. We collectively feel that we've been all over the place emotionally, yet here we are sitting in the same seats in the same room."

After a deliberate pause, the depth of this lesson begins to become clear. Through the activity, I directed their emotional attention to specific events, but the profound lesson of that experience is that we unconsciously do this to ourselves all day, every day, seven days a week, every week of the year, year in and year out. Where we choose to place our emotional attention, every moment of every day, profoundly affects our psychological outlook and physiological reaction patterns. Through those choices, we control how we feel and how we perceive the world in which we live.

This message is at the core of this book. So far, you have read about the physiological processes of how these reaction patterns occur, along with a detailed description of why our emotional reaction patterns are so strongly determined by where we keep our attention. However, experiencing this shift first hand demonstrates the empowering lesson that we have control. During this activity, we *felt* the shift of emotional states by choosing to focus our attention.

An incredible amount of research demonstrates neuroplasticity, or the brain's ability to change through the constant stimulus we provide. That power to change is the underlying theme of this book. However, the lesson that we have the power to change is only half of the message. The other half is that our current patterns of emotional attention are creating our current reaction patterns. We need to realize that our current behaviors of looking for catastrophe, constant negative mental chatter, and willingness to focus on the negative rather than the positive are literally creating who we are right now. We are left with more of the same unless we choose to embrace change. In Chapter Five we begin to examine the power of emotional attention, negative and positive, in the way we live our lives.

The Importance of Emotion

Introduction

In Chapter One, I shared the statement by Lama Surya Das about Tibetan Buddhists' belief that at the heart of every single person is an inner radiance that reflects our essential nature, which is always, utterly positive.[1] I believe that turning inward and tapping into this nature is the only place we will find genuine feelings of gratitude, compassion, love, calm, and connection. I also believe that by sincerely and consistently feeling the presence of those higher emotional states in our lives, we profoundly change who we are and the way we function in the world. One of the most important concepts of this book is how we are biologically changed, which automatically leads to a change in internal coherence, behavior, and inspired productivity, by functioning from those states as opposed to states of anxiety, fear, frustration, or anger.

So far our focus has been on what happens to us physically and psychologically when we function from negative states of feeling. In Chapter Six we will make the transition to examining the transformation that happens when we function from positive states of feeling. However, first we must take a deeper look at the process of specific feeling states, or emotion, as those feeling states are manifest. Antonio Damasio states that the feeling is the mental, private experience of an outwardly observable emotion; therefore, the emotion occurs first.[2] This may be true, but I would also argue that is possible to make a conscious intention to focus on specific feeling states and therefore create specific emotional states, which can change our total way of being.

As we travel further into our metaphorical labyrinth to examine our feeling state as a choice, we will first explore the process of emotion and how those emotions profoundly affect our behavior. That is the focus of this chapter. However, before delving into the process of emotion, let's look at the way emotion has traditionally been treated in research and the overall cultural assumption that emotion, in itself, is something of a weakness. This chapter takes us on the journey from examining the overall concept of emotion, to the process of emotional reaction patterns originating in the limbic system of the brain, to the biochemistry of emotion, and finally to the electrical patterns emanating from our heart, reflecting our breathing patterns and ultimately our emotional state. All of these topics are important considerations on our journey to developing emotional resilience, cultivated higher internal experience, and higher potential by turning inward.

Emotion's Bad Reputation

"You're too emotional!" I heard her say, intending the statement as an insult. "Look at that kid, he's emo!" my son said, and I had to ask him what that meant. He said emo stands for emotional and represents a group of people who wallow in negative emotions. My problem with both of these statements is the powerful underlying assumption that somehow emotion is a bad thing.

Emotion, in my opinion, has gotten a bad rap. In our cognitive-driven society, emotion is seen as a weakness, an obstacle to rational functioning. I also believe it represents a gender bias: Women, on the whole, are seen as too emotional, and men as their rational counterpart. There is a fundamental problem with this line of thinking, however, because the denial of emotion also means the denial of positive emotion. What would our lives be like without love, happiness, or compassion? Additionally, there is ample evidence that positive emotion enhances cognitive functioning and gives meaning to reason. This book presents ample evidence that routinely experiencing higher emotional states is as beneficial to our functioning as human beings as negative emotional reactive states are detrimental.

Additionally, emotion and reason are often seen as opposite ends of a continuum. In reality, as we will find in later chapters, reason becomes less effective without emotion or meaning. One study showed that surgically excising the amygdala also removes the means of meaning—and, therefore, impairs reasoning. We should focus more on the quality and level of emotional state rather than on whether emotion in itself is a good or bad thing. Emotion and cognition constitute a whole human being, and the cultivation of positive emotion may be the missing link in creating whole, happy, and cognitively flourishing lives.

The cultural denial of emotion seems to mirror the denial or reluctance to address the area of emotion in science. As Damasio notes, "Given the magnitude of the matters to which emotion has been attached, one would have expected both philosophy and the sciences of mind and brain to have embraced their study. Surprisingly, that is only happening now."[3] He goes on to state that until quite recently, both neuroscience and cognitive science gave the study of emotion a very cold shoulder.

Neuroscience, or the study of the structure and function of nerve activity in the brain, and cognitive neuroscience are beginning to embrace the study of emotion. Now many are questioning the assumption that emotion and reason are opposites. In addition to the aforementioned study of a removed amygdala, some studies have shown patients who have lost a certain class of emotion through neurological damage also lost their ability to make rational decisions. Damasio suggests that well-targeted and well-deployed emotion seems to be a support system for reason to operate properly. Joseph LeDoux argues that emotion gives meaning to conscious thought.[4]

I truly believe that the question we should be addressing is not whether emotion is a hindrance to cognitive functioning—or more importantly, to the ability to live a productive and happy life—but which types of emotion serve us and which do not. Not only does the word *emotion* have a negative connotation as if it were something to be feared or denied, something that inherently makes us weak, there is almost no recognition that the ability to intentionally cultivate positive emotion, or higher emotional states as in the form of love, compassion, or gratitude, might be the greatest asset we have.

The Meaning and Activation of Emotion

What is emotion? The concept of emotion is quite like the concept of stress, in that the research lacks any universally agreed-upon definition of the term. Neil McNaughton in *Biology and Emotion* states,

> Unfortunately, there has never been any clear agreement as to what the word means. Amongst philosophers, emotion has almost always played an inferior role . . . often as an antagonist to logic and reason. . . . Those who are sure that they know the meaning of the word have often proceeded to experiment without ensuring that what they wish to study is objectively indentifiable. Those who are unsure of its meaning have often attempted to solve the problem by purely linguistic analysis without recourse to experimental data at all.[5]

McNaughton goes on to ask, "If we cannot agree on the meaning of the word, how can we use it objectively?" As an answer to this question, he offers that a biological approach is a good starting point. In addition, he contends that specific emotions might be better defined as the biological response pattern they incur. This approach to defining emotions would separate specific emotions one from another and identify clusters of reaction patterns. "From a biological point of view, which reactions are termed emotional and which are not is far less important than whether we understand the mechanism and function of the reactions and whether we can relate specific reactions to general principles," he argues.[6]

Beginning with a biological point of view, we begin to comprehend how our physiological and psychological reaction patterns determine our behavior, perception, and quality of being. These general principles of reaction give us the tools to be able to cultivate positive reaction patterns. Again, it is emotion that supplies meaning to our lives, and we don't have to fall victim to negative reaction patterns. Intentionally cultivating positive feeling states helps foster positive reactive patterns, which in turn change our way of being.

Our culture seems to subscribe to a belief system that accepts as truth a dichotomy between thinking and feeling, and the feeling state takes a far inferior role. However, when we understand that emotional responses are, for the most part, generated unconsciously[7] and are by far the most powerful biologically, we begin to grasp the unleashed potential of cultivating higher emotional states.

We begin our explanation of the origin of emotion with the limbic system in the brain. Rhawn Joseph states that the limbic system is preeminent in the control and meditation of all aspects of emotion. Additionally, he argues that it is completely capable of overwhelming the "rational" mind because of the massive neural projections leading from the amygdala to the neocortex. That is, our brains lead with emotion and then try to reason, rather than the other way around. Despite all of our evolutionary advances, man remains a creature of emotion.[8]

When we take the way the brain is wired into consideration, it becomes apparent that stress, anxiety, and other negative emotional reactive patterns are primarily distorted reactions. An in-depth look at the development of emotional reactive patterns begins our journey. After we have a conceptual understanding of how these reactive patterns develop, then we begin to explore the possibilities of cultivating those reactive patterns to work for us instead of against us. As Youngey Mingun Rinpoche states, taking the time to gain even a partial understanding of the structure and function of the brain provides a more grounded basis for understanding the dynamics of how and why certain techniques work. He later states, "You are not the limited, anxious person you think you are."[9]

Looking for the Key to Emotion

What makes emotion different from purely conscious thought, and why would this difference be a factor in reducing stress and anxiety, cultivating positive emotion, and transforming our lives? The next section lays the foundation for the process of emotion in the brain. When we begin to comprehend the neural and anatomical differences between emotion and conscious thought, we can better understand and control our negative reaction patterns. Moreover, we begin to understand the shortcomings and inadequacy of transformation through purely conscious thought and get closer to the power of transformation through redirecting our emotional attention to more positive and loving states.

As emotional beings, LeDoux notes, we tend to think of an emotional reaction—be it the experience of stress, anxiety, or the all-consuming feeling of being in love—as a conscious experience. But when we begin to examine the process of emotion in the brain, we see that the conscious experience of that emotion is only part, and not necessarily the most central aspect, of the experience. The most central function, then, is not the conscious awareness of the experience as much as the functions of the systems that generate the emotional experience.[10] In other words, grasping the dynamics of the origination point and the process of emotion is more important in our ability to understand that experience than our conscious reaction to the experience itself. Understanding the reactive process is the key in changing that process.

Like anxiety, emotion originates in a different part of the brain than where we consciously experience it. Have you ever immediately liked or disliked someone and not known why? Have you ever had an immediate and inappropriate anxiety or stressful reaction to something that didn't seem to deserve that reaction? Have you ever had a strong physical and psychological reaction to a circumstance that seemed out of proportion to the specifics of that situation?

We see this concept replayed over and over again in love relationships. How many times have you been in an argument with a partner and felt that he or she was really arguing with some distant previous partner or attaching inappropriate emotional reaction patterns to what was happening in the moment? How many times have you exhibited this type of behavior? How many times have you been overcome with fear, anxiety, jealousy, or insecurity that, on later review, was inconsistent with the severity of the circumstance? Has this type of negative reaction influenced your perception of the event enough that you ended up sabotaging the situation?

I believe that recognizing where negative emotion or emotional unease originates in the brain and the process of these negative emotional reaction patterns is the absolute foundation of being able to change those patterns. Why does anxiety or stress seem to overwhelm us, sometimes to the point that we cannot function? Why, when we are in the depths of difficulty with a loved one, do we recall every similar emotional experience or difficulty we have had with that person or another, when it may not even be relevant to the current experience? Why do we seem to create or re-create the same emotional experiences we fear?

I am convinced that the answers to these questions can be found and ultimately solved by understanding the physiology of the human brain. We need to go to the origination point of emotion to find our key. In demonstrating this concept, I am reminded of the following story: One night a man was frantically searching for his keys under a lamppost. He had dropped them somewhere and desperately needed them to get home. A woman observing his plight asked what was wrong and if she could help. After he explained the situation, she asked where he was standing when he dropped the keys. He pointed to a rosebush about ten feet away. Exasperated, the woman asked why in the world he was looking in this spot instead of where he dropped them. He replied, "The light is better over here." When it comes to the transformation of stress and anxiety and the cultivation of higher emotional states and higher potential, the origination point of emotional experience is where the keys are.

Why Neuroscience?

Biochemistry. Neuroscience. Brain synapse patterns. What do all these have to do with emotion? Understanding the underlying physiology of emotion gives us the foundation for promoting life change through the experience of positive emotion and shows us the damage we are doing to ourselves by choosing to remain stuck. To deny emotion exists is fruitless. To assume that all emotion is negative and something to be controlled loses the phenomenal potential of transformation through the cultivation of higher emotional states. Understanding the physiological processes of emotion gives us the foundation of knowledge necessary to grasp the immense destructive powers of wallowing in negative emotional states and the tremendously powerful possibilities of cultivating higher emotional states.

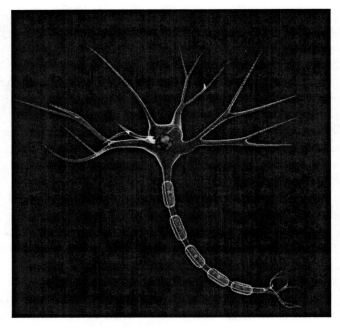

FIGURE 5.1 Diagram of a typical neuron

A Beginner's Guide to the Emotion Process

Although an in-depth description of emotional processing in the brain and body is far beyond the scope of this book, a simplified version suitable for our purposes follows. When we begin to examine emotion, it is important to have a basic understanding of the nervous system and the body's chemistry, or biochemistry, as they relate to psychology. The field of neuroscience is this convergence.

The central nervous system is comprised of the brain and spinal cord. Nerve cells, called neurons, control and primarily constitute this system. Each neuron consists of a cell body, usually one long axon that sends signals and several dendrites that receive signals (Figure 5.1). Neurons can communicate with hundreds of thousands of other neurons through a continuous exchange of information.

An electrical current passes through a nerve when it is activated and a certain type of biochemical called a *neurotransmitter* is released. Neurotransmitters function as signaling substances between two nerve cells or a nerve cell and a target organ. The connection between these, facilitated by the neurotransmitter, is called a *synapse*. When the impulse is sent across the synapse, it is accepted by the receiving nerve cell or organ through a receptor site specifically for that class of neurotransmitters. Once the neurotransmitter occupies the receptor site, it begins a reaction inside the receiving cell.

In addition to neurotransmitters, other chemicals released by cells are called *neurohormones* and *neuropeptides*. While a neurotransmitter crosses the synaptic cleft between nerve cells, neurohormones and neuropeptides are signaling substances simultaneously produced and received throughout the body and brain.[11]

When we have a thought or a feeling, the brain responds by releasing corresponding neurochemicals. These neurochemicals, in the form of neurotransmitters, neurohormones, and mostly neuropeptides, are both produced and received in the brain. What is most important about this process in regard to emotion is that the parts of the brain that are richest in peptides are most involved in the expression of emotion, positive and negative.[12]

In other words, when we have a feeling, we release a cascade of chemical responses throughout our brains and bodies. The parts of the brain that are involved in emotion, namely the limbic system, are richest in the receptor sites for those chemicals. Furthermore, receptor sites for these peptides occur on mobile cells of the immune system, providing a network of chemical communication between the brain and body. According to Candace Pert, these responses probably represent the chemical basis for emotion.[13]

What does all this mean? Every time we have a thought or feeling or interpret something in which we attach meaning, we produce powerful chemicals that activate many cells and organs throughout our body. One of the most affected areas is the emotional center in the brain. This area, the limbic system, then activates a more powerful emotional response. Furthermore, these chemicals are carried throughout our body. Every cell in our body may have 10,000 receptor sites for various neurochemicals.[14]

To underscore this point further, the chemicals that are densely located in the limbic system are largely responsible for information processing in the emotional brain. Such is the circular nature of emotion. Where we place our feeling attention promotes more of the same emotional reaction patterns. These reaction patterns eventually become ingrained response patterns. We are literally training ourselves to respond in a specific way. Where we keep our feeling attention every moment of every day profoundly affects the general nature of how we feel and behave and how we live our lives.

At the most basic level, the chemicals produced through our feeling states and emotional attention eventually dictate who we are at any given moment. Additionally, although neurotransmitters are the chemical substances responsible for the firing of neural nets in the brain, other neurochemicals and hormones likely influence the release and activity of these neurotransmitters. A good example of this is the neurotransmitter dopamine and the hormone oxytocin.

Oxytocin will take center stage in our later discussions of positive emotion, but for now I will use it as a brief example of how specific feeling states create and strengthen neural network firing patterns in our brain. According to Kerstin Uvnas Moberg, a leading researcher on oxytocin, this hormone and the neurotransmitter dopamine are involved in reciprocal patterns of production. In other words, dopamine and other neurotransmitters acting as signaling substances influence the release of oxytocin, and oxytocin, in turn, most likely influences the release and activity of dopamine.[15]

What is significant about this pattern is that oxytocin is known as the bonding hormone and dopamine is a neurotransmitter responsible for the firing of neural networks or brain synapse patterns. The more we bond and create loving connections, the more oxy-tocin we produce, which in turn creates the release and activity of dopamine, which then establishes stronger neural networks for bonding. Remember, any neural network in the brain that repeatedly fires from a specific thought, action, or emotion creates stronger neu-ral networks that allow us to remain in that state or more often function from that state. The more often a specific feeling state or emotion is repeated, the stronger and more long-term is the relationship created in the neural network firing from that state.

This same process is true of negative emotional reaction patterns like anxiety and stress. Think back to our discussion of how anxiety is created and stored in the brain. In our exploration of emotional reaction patterns, we will revisit and expand upon the con-cepts shared in the discussion of anxiety in chapter two. Once these concepts are clear, we will engage in an activity/personal reflection identifying our own damaging emotional reac-tion patterns. Understanding and identifying these destructive patterns is the first step in replacing those patterns with ones conducive to emotional health, well-being, and internal coherence.

As with the man searching for his keys under the lamppost, scientists who try to explain emotion by way of conscious thought and reasoning are looking in the wrong place. The origination point of emotion is where we must begin, as this is where our subcon-scious reactive patterns are stored. This is also where there is hope of intentionally chang-ing those reactive patterns. Again, in the explanation of emotional experience, we will use as a foundation the discussion of the development and experience of anxiety presented in Chapter Two. Much of the ensuing conversation of the dynamics of emotional experience draws heavily on the work of Joseph LeDoux, arguably the world's leading researcher on fear and emotion.

When we examine the dynamics of emotion, the first question is whether emotion is always a conscious experience. If it is not, what is the relevance of a subconscious emo-tional experience? To analyze this question, we must first remember our primary goal in studying emotion. It is my contention that stress and anxiety cut us off from our internal selves and that operating from the love, care, and compassion residing within each one of us automatically and physiologically reduces that stress and anxiety. So, what does the study of emotion have to do with all of this? And what is the power in intentionally culti-vating higher emotional states?

At its core, stress is a feeling of emotional unease. This unease may be associated with a particular stressor, a general set of stressors, or a free floating feeling of anxiety, but this physi-cal feeling state of being emotionally uneasy most accurately characterizes what we experi-ence. Simply put, we don't feel well. If the physical feeling of emotional unease characterizes stress, we need to take a careful look at the origination point of those physical feelings.

To do so, we need to consider the working of the limbic system, specifically the amyg-dala, implicit vs. explicit memory, the definition and specifics of emotional memory, the ingredients of the process of emotional memory and conscious experience, and the recogni-tion of triggers of reactive behavior. Only then can we begin to replace negative reactive behavior and feelings of physical and psychological unease with intentionally cultivated feelings of internal coherence or higher emotional states. As you will see, there is much

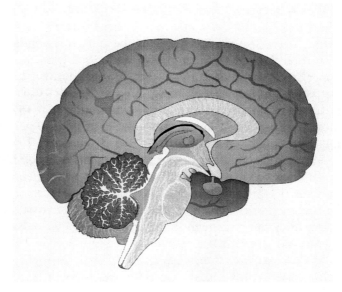

FIGURE 5.2   A split view of the inside of the brain. This diagram shows a distinct difference between the outer cortex, or the "thinking" part of the brain, and the limbic or emotional inner centers of the brain.

more to emotional experience then what meets the mind's eye, and emotional feelings involve much more of the brain that does thought or conscious experience. Remember LeDoux's contention that emotions give meaning to thought.[16]

Initially what we learned about the dynamics of emotion came from split-brain surgery in the 1970s. Split-brain surgery was a procedure that severed nerve connections between the two hemispheres of the brain in an attempt to control severe epilepsy. Because the hemispheres of the brain are responsible for different tasks and severing the connections between hemispheres cuts off communication between them, we began to see a psychological dichotomy between thinking and feeling.[17] When examining stress and emotion, if we don't consider the feeling states and physiological reactions of those states, we are looking in the wrong place.

From the discoveries of the split-brain theory, it became clear that a feeling, or the physiological arousal from that feeling, did not have to involve conscious awareness, which is processed by the left hemisphere. In other words, we don't have to be consciously aware that we're having an emotional reaction to exhibit its physical and psychological consequences. Additionally, even though emotional feelings may be subconsciously activated, the physiological responses they incur can be objectively measured. Thinking and feeling are two distinct states, but the feeling state of emotional experience can be measured without input of conscious awareness; therefore, it must come from a separate system in the brain. LeDoux's work amazingly showed that neural pathways for feelings bypass the neocortex, the thinking part of the brain.

Where do feelings originate? This question brings us back to the limbic system and more specifically the amygdala. In *Emotional Intelligence*, Daniel Goleman says the amygdala is the specialist for emotional matters and tells the story of a young man who had his amygdala removed to control severe seizures. Afterward, he was perfectly capable of conversation, but he no longer recognized close friends and relatives, not even his mother. "Without an amygdala he seemed to have lost all recognition of feeling," Goleman notes, adding that the amygdala acts as a storehouse of emotional memory. It is solely responsible for determining significance; thus, life without an amygdala is stripped of personal meanings.[18]

Emotional memory comes up frequently in our discussion of emotion. It is very important at this point that the definition of emotional memory is completely clear. Emotional memory differs from cognitive or conscious memory in that emotional memory is implicit. Implicit memories and explicit memories carry with them a very different physiological process. Explicit memories are conscious recollections, or those things that we can consciously remember. They can be brought to mind and described verbally.[19]

An implicit memory, or emotional memory, involves implicit or unconscious processes and does not depend on conscious awareness. I like to refer to implicit memories as our subconscious reactive patterns, a whole body feeling reaction in response to something often beyond conscious awareness. Again, when we experience a negative emotional memory, we have a biochemical and neural rush throughout our body, and we feel a sense of unease. As in our discussion of anxiety, once this learning about a specific stimulus has occurred, the new stimulus doesn't even have to be consciously perceived to elicit a response, or it may even be just a remote replica of the original event, not deserving the emotional response we attribute to it. Our amygdala has stored conditioned emotional responses or reactive patterns to a phenomenal number of stimuli, and these reactive patterns need only be vaguely familiar to elicit the conditioned response.

For instance, I may have had an experience sometime in my life of feeling inadequate. That conditioned emotional reactive pattern, or emotional memory, is stored in my amygdala. Anytime any circumstance carries a remote resemblance to that feeling, my conditioned emotional patterns are released, and throughout my body biochemical and neural messages are sent as if it were the first time I experienced this threat. Neither the initial experience nor subsequent circumstances require conscious awareness.

Usually, our feeling reaches conscious awareness. At that point, it becomes subjective. Our bodies feel this feeling, or physiological reaction, and our brains want to make sense of it. Unfortunately, because most of us don't understand this process, we quite often mistakenly attach the conditioned emotional response to what we are experiencing at the moment to the current event to validate our feeling state. In essence, we become victims to our negative reactive patterns because we feel they are always justified by the current circumstance. Even if they are justified, falling victim to our own reactive patterns only makes us less able to clearly and coherently deal with the event. LeDoux contends our conscious experience of the emotion, and not the emotional experience itself, is the problem.[20]

This reactive pattern was developed through evolution for a purpose. As our species developed, it was important to be drawn toward the things that would allow our species to continually prosper and turned away from those things that would threaten our survival.

Since the amygdala gives meaning or significance to a thought or event, its activation sends a systemwide biochemical and neural alert to what it has perceived. The fundamental point is that this alert is experienced as a physiological and psychological feeling throughout our bodies, immediate and without conscious intent.

This system may serve an important role in warning us of potentially dangerous situations. The reactive patterns may not always be misplaced and may even serve as a good monitor for what is healthy or not healthy. The key lies in awareness. If we notice or observe our own reactions to specific stimuli without getting caught up in them, we can decide whether our reactive patterns are appropriate for those circumstances. Additionally, if we can disengage from the automatic negative reactive pattern by replacing it with a positive pattern, we can take concrete steps to deal with the situation from an emotionally coherent place.

Before exploring how all this information can be used for positive transformation, let's briefly review how our emotional trigger points are created and then honestly and genuinely examine our own trigger points. Self-understanding of the process of our own conditioned responses and trigger points is a necessary step to move beyond being held hostage by our personal reactive patterns.

Emotional Trigger Points

When we have an emotional experience, positive or negative, our reactive patterns are automatically activated. Conscious awareness and processing of the experience doesn't happen until the stimulus that originated in the amygdala reaches the cortex, or thinking part of the brain. Then we begin to reason and process the experience. An important point to remember is that there are more neural projections leading from the amygdala to the cortex than from the cortex to the amygdala. *What this means is that our emotional reactive response is stronger and quicker than our ability to reason that response.*

The amygdala also sends signals of heightened awareness to the cortex, most often throwing the brain's electrical patterns out of sync. In addition to the stimulation of electrical patterns in the brain, neurotransmitters and other chemicals are released for heightened awareness. Normally this process is advantageous as cortical arousal makes us more alert in memory, perception, and problem solving. The problem is when we get too much arousal, we become overanxious and unproductive. Strong emotional reactions are most often involved in cortical over-arousal.

A final point to remember is that the amygdala activates our whole body by way of the autonomic nervous system, hormonal system, organs, and glands. This activation sends profound chemical, electrical, and energetic reactions throughout whole body, which in turn sends impulses back to the brain that serve to perpetuate that cycle. All of these reactions work in concert to determine the way we consciously feel at any given time.

Shortly we will examine how there is transformative power in understanding this process and how cultivating positive or higher emotional feeling states through conscious intent can make this process work for us. First, though, we must examine our own stress and anxiety trigger points in this process. To do so, we must remember several facts. When this process is related to stress or anxiety as in a negative emotional reaction, it can be released independent of and prior to thought. This response sends a systemwide physiological and psychological reaction throughout our bodies and brains. Sometimes it is consciously processed, but sometimes it is not. Quite often the conscious processing of the reactive pattern is faulty and we ascribe the intense emotional reaction of unease to whatever situation is currently in our awareness. In other words, our reaction may be far out of proportion to the circumstance, and our reactive patterns may cloud our perception of the severity of the current circumstance.

What is most important to remember when we begin the transformation process is that stress and anxiety are feeling reactions. We feel the enormous physiological effects throughout our body. The electrical impulses in the brain and heart get out of sync, the body is loaded with biochemical reactions, and accordingly, the brain responds with a perception of stress. All these reactions powerfully affect the way we consciously feel, both psychologically and physically. These are learned triggers of defensive behavior.[21]

Recognizing the physical reaction of your stress and anxiety response is the first step in identifying your personal triggers. If you have a strong physical reaction in similar or like circumstances, this is probably a trigger for you. Sometimes it takes looking closely to find a thread connecting some of your triggers. Common examples are underlying feelings of inadequacy, guilt, rejection, or needing to be perfect. This feeling state may replay itself in a variety of circumstances. If you can recognize the response by identifying the physical feeling, you can begin to take responsibility for, and ultimately reduce, your triggers for that implicit emotional reactive pattern.

Identifying Your Personal Trigger Points
EXERCISE AND REFLECTION # 3

Understanding how negative emotional memory is stored and consequently activated by the brain is the first step in being able to take control of these response patterns. After reading the section on the development, storage, and activation of emotional memory, process and reflect on situations in your own life where this psycho-physiological process is likely to occur. The more successful you are at identifying your own trigger points, large and small, the more successful you are likely to be in growing out of this paralyzing pattern and taking control of your emotional resilience. We all have these triggers. Some may be subtle and hidden, or you may be consciously aware that you have strong reactions to specific circumstances.

This exercise requires humility and a genuine willingness to examine and take responsibility for your response patterns. The nature of the emotional memory reaction pattern is to blame whatever situation is currently present for the emotional reaction we are having. Take notice when a negative emotional reaction pattern feels familiar, as in these examples:

"You're just like my former partner."

"I always freeze up on important tests or interviews."

"I hate it when someone criticizes me or gets angry or disappointed with me."

Also, pay attention to the more subtle reactions you experience. Do you get a "knot" in your stomach in response to some situations? Do you get a vague feeling of threat or emotional unease in circumstances that carry a similar underlying theme? Pay attention to both the psychological and physiological reaction you experience.

If a specific negative feeling state recurs or often replays itself in various circumstances, there is a strong chance that feeling state is stored as negative emotional memory and possibly activated at inappropriate times. The activation of this negative response pattern sends a cascade of negative emotional reaction patterns throughout the body and brain and greatly diminishes our ability to perceive and react to the current situation in an emotionally appropriate manner. Again, these response patterns may be large or small, but both cause significant unease. The seemingly less-significant patterns may cause lasting problems because we are reluctant to recognize them.

Three possibilities may account of the recurrence of a negative emotional reaction:

1. An emotional memory trigger is activated and the current situation, while possibly uncomfortable, does not warrant the negative emotional reaction we ascribe to it, which severely inhibits our ability to perceive and react in a positive, constructive, or appropriate manner.

91

2. The situation needs to be acted upon, but fear and anxiety are paralyzing states. Redirecting our emotional attention to a higher emotional state will help us more constructively and clearly deal with the situation.

3. We subconsciously draw situations or people into our lives with similar negative circumstances because these circumstances invoke personal issues we need to deal with constructively and move beyond for our own personal growth.

The attributes of these situations may overlap, but taking responsibility for our emotional recurrence is the only way to effectively grow through this process and eliminate the victim attitude that often accompanies these recurrences. We need to be authentic and truthful about our reaction patterns, for this is the only way to true growth. Additionally, these reaction patterns may manifest in more of a passive state. A recurring pattern that I have had to work hard to grow through is finding my voice.

This is a much more subtle pattern for me, but it has held throughout a good portion of my life. As the youngest of five children and taking into account some of the dynamics that set me apart from my siblings as a group, I learned it wasn't OK for me to stand out. I learned to hide my voice for fear of standing out, and I have had to work hard to overcome the anxiety reaction I get when I know I need to grow or develop in a certain way by speaking up for myself. This anxiety reaction is relatively mild and carries a general sense of unease.

One of my more obvious triggers, but still damaging and reactive, is a strong knot in my stomach and tightness in my chest when I am exposed to any situation that brings up feelings of abandonment. Because this is a universal theme for me, it can replay itself in many different circumstances. I have learned to first identify it by the physical feeling reaction, by noticing how my body and emotions respond to specific situations.

What sets you off? What situations or circumstances seem to elicit a predictable response in you? Keep in mind that these trigger points manifest themselves in physical, sometimes strong, reactions. Many times we are conscious first of the physical feeling, but sometimes we are so accustomed to these physical response patterns that we don't consciously notice them. We just feel awful and begin to unconsciously ascribe psychological reactions that may or may not be appropriate. Notice physical response patterns to stressful situations. What situations in your life cause strong physical reactions? Review "The Feeling States of Stress" worksheet. Where in your body do you usually feel stressful reactions? Use these reaction patterns as a guide to your potential trigger points.

Honestly list and describe several personal, professional, or academic situations where negative emotional response patterns recur for you. These response patterns usually carry a definite physiological reaction or feeling state. List the trigger points and the typical physical reaction you get with them. If you are having trouble understanding this concept, reflect on certain situations or circumstances that "set you off" emotionally. Be honest. Look for themes and patterns. Be authentic and genuine—sometimes examining the situations that seem to set you off provides valuable information about your personal trigger points.

After listing and describing situations where negative emotional response patterns recur, as honestly as possible examine whether this response pattern has become part of your negative emotional memory, a repeat of circumstances you need to grow through, or both. Reflect and process. How can you best deal with these negative response patterns when they occur? How can you take responsibility that the emotional reaction to the event is yours and may cloud your perception of the event itself? How can you "own" these response patterns? If something replays for you over and over, it may be something that you need to learn to recognize. How can you recognize these situations as trigger points and still objectively deal with the current situation?

_____

_____

_____

_____

_____

_____

_____

_____

_____

_____

_____

_____

It is also of paramount importance to remember that the situations may warrant action on your part. However, recognizing the physical reactive pattern and disengaging from the physical response are the first steps in being able to deal with the situation in a less reactive and more emotionally stable way. In Chapter Ten we will discuss semantics in dealing with situations in a less emotionally reactive state, and in Chapter Eleven we will begin to discuss how to take appropriate external action from a caring, compassionate, kind, and empowered emotional state. For now, it is important to train yourself to identify your own reactive patterns.

The Mood Congruency Hypothesis

The mood congruency hypothesis states that our current mood state determines the emotional memory response patterns activated deep within our brains. As we will note in later chapters, sometimes the best course of action is to remove yourself from the situation, reset your own emotional physiology, and return to the situation in a more coherent and clear emotional state. A thorough grasp of the mood congruency hypothesis provides a more complete understanding of the damaging effects of allowing yourself to get carried away or wallow in negative reactive states.

When we are in specific mood, feeling, or emotional state, we seem to be only able to feel more of that same state. Have you ever been in an argument with someone and suddenly everything he or she has ever done to make you angry resurfaces? Or have you been in a situation that reminds you of a similar event that upset you in the past and all those negative memories resurface? Have you had situations when all your emotional attention is on fear of failure and all your present thoughts become focused on all your past failures?

Mood congruity of memory, or the mood congruency hypothesis, states that recall of specific memories is more acute when a person is in the same mood state as that memory.[22] It is true that we are more likely to have unpleasant memories when we are sad, and depressed people seem only capable of depressive memories. Another idea, called state dependent recall, holds that we are much more capable of remembering learned information when we are in the same mood state as we were when we originally learned that information. This type of recall has powerful implications and will be explored further in the next chapter. For now, let's focus on the concept that where we have our emotional attention perpetuates more of the same emotional memory, implicit and explicit.

The mood congruency hypothesis holds that our current mood state determines the emotional memory, or emotional reactive patterns activated deep within the brain. Some scientists theorize that memory is stored in associative networks and specific conditions are more likely to activate these networks. One of the most important conditions in activating specific associative memory networks is the current emotional state you are experiencing, whether implicit (emotional reaction feelings) or explicit (conscious memory). In other words when we feel depressed, all we can think of is all the things that are wrong; when we are angry, all we can think of is all the things about which we have a right to be angry. When we are overwhelmed or anxious, all we can think of is all the pressures facing us. Conversely, when we are in love, "in the zone," or functioning from higher emotional states, all we can think about is the positive side of specific situations.

R. Joseph maintains that so much emotional memory is stored in the amygdala it is actually a safety mechanism to be able to process only similar emotional reaction patterns at one time. He argues that if the information were not filtered to maintain one emotional reality at a time, our system would be completely overwhelmed with competing streams of input.[23] As we begin to comprehend the importance of understanding emotional memory and emotional reactive patterns, it also becomes apparent that paying attention to our current mood state is of paramount importance in developing internal coherence.

If our emotional memories come up as feeling reactive patterns, and we choose to stay in those states longer than serves us—by wallowing in those patterns, castrophizing, retelling and recreating those same issues—the mood congruency hypothesis tells us we will create more of those same reactive patterns. We call up any explicit memory that matches that mood state, and we expose ourselves to all the physiological damage and negative adaptations associated with that mood state. Knowledge about this process is power. Intentional cultivation of mood states based on gratitude, care, compassion, and love is even greater power. Now we move on to discuss effective ways to stop the destructive process of stress, anxiety, and emotional unease and begin a process of higher emotional states, empowering potential, and inner harmony.

The Power of Disengaging from the Negative

The rest of this chapter focuses on recognizing and disengaging from our negative reactive patterns. In Chapter Six we will begin to look at the power of cultivating positive emotional states that simultaneously come from the peace and radiance of our internal selves. Through their presence, these states increase internal coherence and higher internal experience. Through our understanding of the biological processes of the body, we realize that we don't have to be the anxious limited person we think we are and understand that we can create a whole different and empowered way of being.

In *The Joy of Living: Unblocking the Secrets and Science of Happiness,* Yongey Mingyour Rinpoche states that most people simply mistake the habitually formed, neuron-constructed image of themselves for who and what they really are.[24] So far, we have focused on how we construct those neuronal images. Now it is time to examine how we grow beyond those images. As we look at that potential for growth, we need to consider first how to disengage from those destructive images.

In the disengagement process, it is important to be able to identify our negative feeling reactive patterns and not become victims to those patterns. Among the many terms that have been used for this process are "become the observer" or "cultivate the witness." This is an important step because if we are not consciously aware that these are our reactive patterns, we may mistake them for our prescribed reality. Later we will venture into the realm of replacing those negative reactive patterns with life-enhancing reactive patterns, but the first step is recognizing and disengaging from our life-depleting negative reactive patterns.

In returning our discussion to conscious vs. subconscious emotional reactive patterns, it is important to remember that even though the origination point of the reactive response is subconscious, the feeling usually becomes conscious at some point. The problem with this scenario is that although the feeling becomes conscious, we may not be aware of it. In other words, we may be consciously feeling bad or full of unease, but that feeling may not be the center of our awareness. When we are not fully aware of these patterns, we are more likely to ascribe circumstances to be responsible for the feeling instead of our own personal reactive patterns.

LeDoux states that emotional feelings result when we become consciously aware that an emotion system in the brain is active.[25] When we become consciously aware of this feeling, we automatically want to ascribe a subjective, psychological feeling to that reaction and then justify that feeling: we feel bad, we feel upset, we feel angry or hurt. Overall reactive patterns then become exacerbated or made worse because we feel entitled to be the victim of these subjective feelings, which may even become "you make me angry," "you hurt me," or "you upset me."

The first step in disengaging from this process is to become consciously aware of the physical or psychological feeling and at the same time recognize it as part of our reactive mechanism. By "cultivating the witness" or "becoming the observer," we recognize the reactive process as it occurs but do not get caught up in perpetuating the cycle by assigning subjective meaning to it. I like to call this step "take notice." This process will be discussed in more detail in Chapter Seven as a tool for developing inner harmony.

When we develop the skill of taking notice, we begin to "own" our reaction patterns. This skill requires acute awareness of our physical reaction patterns in response to emotion. Back in the second exercise for reflection, you wrote how you physically felt during a time of stress or anxiety and identified where in your body you felt the reactive pattern. At that time the lesson was to demonstrate how the body is profoundly affected by stress, anxiety, and emotional reactive patterns. Now that same concept can be used to identify when your physical reactive patterns are taking place. If you are not aware that these reactions are taking place, you cannot disengage from them or realize when your subjective interpretation of events is out of balance with the situation.

Where in your body are your typical negative reactive patterns felt? Remember if you are already feeling the reactive patterns in your body, the process of the response has already been activated, although you may only become conscious of it slowly, if at all. Do you tense up? Do you feel a knot in your stomach? Does your chest tighten and your breathing become shallower? There are many possible physical reactive patterns; only you can identify those that activate in you.

The key is in awareness, in taking notice. The key is in learning to catch the reactive pattern as it starts as a physical or psychological reaction, recognize that it is all part of the inborn process described earlier, and then disengage from the subjective judgment of that reactive pattern. Always tune into your bodily reaction patterns as the initial stimulus rather than a result of an already validated psychological feeling.

Learn to identify the physical and psychological feeling as your trigger points. Learn to recognize them as soon as they are activated, witness them, and disengage from them. From there you can replace those feelings with intentionally cultivated feelings of internal peace and make a reasoned reaction to act based on the clear facts rather than from the cloud of negative emotion.

Two things happen when you consistently practice this kind of awareness. The first is that you retrain your reactive patterns; much will be said about that process in the next two chapters. The other is that, after continual practice, your body becomes less reactive and gets much better at identifying the negative reactive patterns when they happen. You immediately notice them because now these patterns more the exception than the rule, and you are used to functioning from a calmer, more emotionally coherent state. Soon you will find you don't like feeling physically upset. You will learn to immediately identify when these patterns begin to be activated and automatically shift to a state of awareness and disengagement from the subjective emotion. Then you can effectively reason an appropriate response.

Being aware of your personal reactive patterns is the first step in being able to identify them for what they are, to let them go, and to make a conscious rational decision about how to proceed.

Exploring Physical Reactive Patterns
EXERCISE AND REFLECTION # 4

Tune into your body. Write and reflect about what you think your physical reactive patterns are. Think about a time when you feel you were exhibiting an emotional reactive pattern and identify specifically where you felt it in your body. Do these physical reactive patterns give you extra information about what your anxiety triggers might be? In other words, reflect how you physically feel in certain situations. Does becoming aware of your physical reaction patterns during certain situations give you additional information on whether those situations might be anxiety trigger points for you? How can you use this information specifically to make concrete change? How can you remind yourself to disengage from this physical reaction?

Write about specific situations where you feel a clear physical reaction. These might seem to be random events, but look for an underlying connection point. Write, process, reflect, and explore the concepts in this chapter. How do they apply to you and how can you use them to begin to notice and disengage from the subjective emotional response you usually experience? Add any reflective thoughts about this process for you and how you can integrate this information into your daily life.

_____

_____

_____

_____

_____

_____

_____

_____

Positive vs. Negative Emotion
EXERCISE AND REFLECTION # 5

I quite often struggle with the idea of emotion as one coherent concept. The enormous psychological and physiological differences between positive and negative emotion, and how these two states determine who we become, are so vast it is hard to ascribe one meaning to the word. Being in love, in the zone, or authentically happy is vastly different than being profoundly depressed, consumed by hatred, or wrought with anxiety. The psychological, physiological, and biochemical states produced by these diverse feeling states are also immensely different. Furthermore, there has never been any clear agreement as to the definition of the concept of emotion.

The premise of this book is that the cultivation of higher emotional feeling states can profoundly affect our bodies, our brains, and our lives. Where we keep our emotional attention or feeling state every moment of every day determines who we become. To internalize the power of this premise, we need to let go of the idea that the concept of emotion in totality is inherently bad or something to be denied. As McNaughton suggested, maybe the best way to define emotion is by the biological response a specific emotion or group of emotions generates.[26] If we define emotions by the type of biological response they generate, there is a very clear-cut distinction between the tremendous power of higher emotional states and the alarmingly detrimental impact of negative emotional states.

Assuming the biological approach and cognizant of the neuroplasticity of the brain in response to what we routinely expose it, intentionally cultivating higher emotional states may be as enormously beneficial as wallowing in negative emotional states is destructive. The question, therefore, is not the definition of emotion as a whole, but which specific emotions elicit a positive biological response in each one of us.

Brainstorm on the following page. Below the line write as many emotional reactions, or feeling states, that elicit a negative physiological reaction for you—simply put, those feelings that make you feel bad.

Above the line brainstorm and write as many emotional reaction or feeling states that elicit a positive physiological reaction, or make you feel good.

As you develop this list, try to identify the words by intensity and emotional level. In other words, list the emotions that elicit the most positive feelings for you highest on the paper and the most negative feelings the lowest. For instance, below the line, I would list hatred, worry, anxiety, fear, insecurity, and guilt. Above the line I would write peacefulness, serenity, compassion, love, caring, kindness, gratitude, and spiritual feelings. Then I would rank these emotions in some sort of hierarchy based on how they affect me.

Emotional Charting

List higher emotional states here

List lower emotional states here

Reflect and Process

Process and reflect on what you wrote. Examine the higher emotional states you listed and why these states stood out in importance for you. For example, after I completed my chart, I would only focus on the higher emotional states I listed and reflect why, for me, these states reflect my chosen higher emotions—simply put, why they mean something to me.

_____

_____

_____

_____

_____

_____

_____

_____

_____

_____

_____

_____

_____

REFERENCES

1. Das, L. S., *Awakening the Buddha Within: Tibetan Wisdom for the Western World* (New York: Broadway Books, 1997).

2. Damasio, A., *The Feeling of What Happens: Body and Emotions in the Making of Consciousness* (San Diego, CA: Harcourt, 1999).

3. Ibid., 42.

4. LeDoux, J., *The Emotional Brain: The Mysterious Underpinnings of Emotional Life* (London: Orion Books, 1998).

5. McNaughton, N., *Biology and Emotion* (Cambridge, Great Britain: Cambridge University Press, 1989): 1.

6. Ibid., 1.

7. LeDoux, J., *The Emotional Brain: The Mysterious Underpinnings of Emotional Life* (New York: Simon and Schuster, 1996).

8. Joseph, R., ed. *Neurotheology: Brain, Science, Spirituality, Religious Experience* (San Jose, CA: University Press, 2003).

9. Rinpoche, Y. M., *The Joy of Living: Unblocking the Secrets and Science of Happiness* (New York: Crown Publishing, 2007): 46.

10. LeDoux, *Emotional Brain*, 1998.

11. Pert, C., *Molecules of Emotion: The Science behind Mind-Body Medicine* (New York: Scribner, 1997).

12. Ibid.

13. Ibid.

14. Ibid.

15. Uvnas Moberg, K., *The Oxytocin Factor: Tapping the Hormone of Love, Calm, and Healing* (Cambridge, MA: Perseus, 2003).

16. LeDoux, *Emotional Brain*, 1998.

17. Ibid.

18. Goleman, D., *Emotional Intelligence: Why It Can Matter More than I.Q.* (New York: Bantam, 1994).

19. LeDoux, J., *The Synaptic Self: How Our Brains Become Who We Are* (New York: Viking, 2002).

20. LeDoux, *Emotional Brain*, 1996.

21. Ibid.

22. Ibid.

23. Joseph, R., *The Transmitter to God: The Limbic System, The Soul, and Spirituality* (San Jose, CA: University Press, 2001).

24. Rinpoche, *Joy of Living.*

25. LeDoux, *Emotional Brain,* 1998.

26. McNaughton, *Biology and Emotion.*

CHAPTER SIX

A Look at the Positive

Introduction to the Positive

The study of emotion has long been ignored, even shunned, by the field of cognitive science. For many years researchers have given much more attention to the cognitive aspects of the brain than those dealing with emotion. Emotion has traditionally been disregarded as an acceptable research subject, and when it has been studied, scientists have focused on its negative context. Researchers have studied the damaging effects of negative emotion, with the apparent assumption that reducing negative affect would necessarily produce a positive emotional response.

Studying emotion does present some challenges. To group the whole class of negative emotions with positive emotions loses the tremendous possibilities of the power of cultivating the positive. To group these emotional states literally takes opposites and treats them as if they are one, downplaying the tremendous impact of emotions at both ends of the spectrum. To presume that studying and subsequently reducing negative emotion automatically results in physiological and psychological benefits in the magnitude of those created by positive emotion is a faulty assumption. Taking steps to reduce negative emotion is only half the story.

At this point in our journey, again using the labyrinth as a metaphor, we are approaching the center. We have learned what stress and anxiety are and how the effects of these states cut us off from the development of our internal selves. We have discovered how the brain processes emotion and examined all the negative biochemical and neural effects that result from negative emotional reactions. We have examined our own trigger points of emotional unease and how these states specifically and individually affect each of us. Finally, we have given particular focus to identifying our physical reaction patterns as a gauge to when we are experiencing ingrained negative reactive patterns.

Now we begin to make the shift. We begin to turn inward. Only recently has research begun to accumulate showing the power of cultivating and routinely experiencing positive emotion. The power within comes from understanding and reducing negative emotional reaction patterns and from turning inward to tap into our vast stores of higher emotions. It comes from conscious intent to make the physiological, neural, and biochemical process of emotion work for us instead of against us.

The focus of this chapter is on making the transition from staying stuck in negative emotional patterns, those filled with stress and anxiety, to intentionally cultivating positive and higher emotional patterns. It is on the remarkable physiological, biochemical, and neural effects of teaching ourselves to routinely feel positive emotional states. It is about the neuroplasticity of the brain under advantageous circumstances and how we can consciously and intentionally promote those circumstances by feeling higher emotions.

To maintain that focus, we will review specific research encouraging the study of positive emotion and what some of those studies have found. This chapter includes specifics on the biochemical process of higher emotions, particularly those of oxytocin, which in recent years has been shown to be connected to a whole host of positive psychological and physiological states. It revisits the process of emotional learning in the brain and how that emotional learning can be transformed through routine experience of higher emotion. It reveals the unique relationship of the amygdala and the electrical patterns of the heart, especially under conditions of higher emotional expression. Finally, it discloses how routine mental and emotional training can bring about significant changes in the structure and function of the human brain, thus profoundly affecting our perception and quality of life.

The Study of Negative and Positive Emotion

Beginning in the 1940s, research in psychology primarily focused on reducing psychological disorder, thus ignoring psychological research with positive intent. Research in the area of emotion has focused on the negative effects of emotion and how to reduce those effects, with no emphasis on intentionally creating positive emotional states. The term affect, when used as a noun, refers to an emotional state or mood; research is beginning to question the assumption that reducing negative emotion will automatically result in positive affect.

The more general field of psychology is also making this shift. According to Mihaly Csikszentmihalyi, a leading researcher in the field of positive psychology, major psychological theories are changing to support the study of a new science of strength and resilience. "No longer do the dominant theories view the individual as a passive vessel responding to stimuli," he notes in support of his contention that this new focus of psychology will be on making normal people stronger, more productive, and able to achieve higher potential.[1] Seligman and Csikszentmihalyi state: "Our message is to remind our field that psychology is not just the study of pathology, weakness, and damage; it is also the study of strength and virtue. Treatment is not just fixing what is broken; it is nurturing what is best."[2] The field of positive psychology validates the study and cultivation of higher emotional states.

Other research supports the notion that to develop the positive we must focus on the positive. MacLeod and Moore argue that positive and negative aspects of experience are actually two separate psychological systems instead of opposite ends of one continuum, and they contend that to develop the positive, we need to focus on the positive. They also argue that intervention through positive psychological focus is an important avenue to develop emotional resilience and that the processing of specific positive experience will increase the chance of a positive affective shift. Finally, MacLeod and Moore recommend tools for a positive affective shift, including identifying and interrupting thoughts that interrupt well-being, mindful awareness, and cognitive therapy with the focus on positive experience.[3] The Higher Emotion and Refocusing Techniques (HEART) presented in Chapter Seven combine these recommendations and synthesize the scientific concepts presented in this book in a usable and practical format.

The MacLeod and Moore and Csikszentmihalyi research is in agreement that to develop positive emotion and cultivate emotional resilience we need to make positive emotion our primary focus, not just aim to reduce the negative. Avia echoes this sentiment and argues that because interventions to reduce negative thinking may not automatically result in a positive affect, we need to seriously consider the study of positive emotions.[4] The new discipline of positive psychology advocates study of the positive to make people stronger, more productive, and able to reach higher potential. The field of stress management has not gotten the message.

Most in the field of stress management still focus on reducing or trying to get rid of stress instead of replacing it. When we focus only on reducing the stress, we are not necessarily creating a positive, more productive and healthy lifestyle. Additionally, anything we focus on will likely persist. The field of stress management can learn from the field of positive psychology. If stress and anxiety are defined as emotional unease, then the absolute best way to relieve that unease is to replace it with cultivated higher emotional states.

I am reminded of a story and a metaphor. The metaphor goes something like this: if I tell you not to think of a yellow kangaroo, what comes immediately to your mind? More than likely, you imagine a yellow kangaroo. If I tell you to instead think of a blue elephant, it is easier to make that shift. If we focus on our stress and anxiety as a way to reduce those states, they remain our main focus. If we create an intentional conscious shift to higher emotional states, it is much easier to maintain them as our focus and that focus automatically reduces our stress and anxiety. This chapter examines the scientific and physiological basis of how that happens.

The story I am reminded of is the one shared earlier about the man searching for his keys under the lamppost when he dropped them somewhere else. The true key in reducing emotional unease is to replace it with another emotional state. We need to look beyond the places traditional stress management programs have shown us. We need to look where the key is, not where we have been unsuccessfully looking.

Making the Mood Congruency Hypothesis Work for Us

Chapter Five introduced the mood congruency hypotheses and discussed how our focused emotional attention stimulates increased biochemical and neural responses that perpetuate more of that same state.[5] To support this point further, Rhawn Joseph states that we have such an enormous amount of emotional reactive memory stored in our brains that our brains can only process like emotional reactions at one time to avoid being overloaded.[6] If the yellow kangaroo represents negative emotional states or emotional unease, and all we are focused on is the yellow kangaroo, that creature will keep showing us for us.

To take this point further, if we can consciously and intentionally create a feeling shift in our bodies and brains, therefore activating the emotional centers in the brain to higher emotional states, those states are activated and perpetuated as our way of being. Additionally, research has shown that cultivating a more positive mood state is associated with more pleasant perception and attention of emotional information than a negative mood state.[7] LeDoux suggests that activating a specific emotion node and experiencing and feeling the relevant emotion activates attention, perception, memory, interpretation, and judgment relevant to that emotion.[8] The power lies with the cultivation of higher emotional states.

Mood Congruency and Cognition

To take the mood congruency hypothesis even further, one study examined personality traits as they relate to mood state. Generally, neuroticism—that is, a depressive or anxious personality trait—was associated with negative cognition, or not being able to think clearly. Conversely, extroversion, or interest and involvement in people or things outside of the self, was associated with positive cognition. In other words, those who were more depressed or anxious were not able to perform as well on tasks to measure their cognitive ability as those who felt better about themselves. This correlation held true when the subjects were in a natural mood state. However, when mood was controlled, this was not the case.[9]

These are fundamentally important findings when examining cognition and emotion. Although personality characteristics may superficially denote a predetermined outcome in our ability to perform mentally, their significance is diminished when mood is controlled. In other words, if a person with personality traits resembling those identified in neuroticism were to approach an anxiety-producing task in a natural mood, this research indicates he or she is likely to have a negative perception and interpretation of the task. Thus, this task becomes a perceived stressor, with the resultant anxiety-driven physiological responses. If this same person were able to shift to a positive emotional state, the results would likely be positive cognition, perception, and interpretation. This research indicates that higher emotional refocusing would likely reduce the negative perception of this event as a stressor, along with the psychological and physiological consequences of that perception. An induced higher emotional mood state may, in fact, be the most appropriate intervention to reduce anxiety in those with negative personality traits.

What does all this mean? It means that those who tend to exhibit negative personality traits, like depression, anxiety, and the like, are more likely to see a task as overwhelming and are more likely to perform poorly. It also means that if these same people could refocus their emotional attention and mood, they would view the task as easier and perform better.

Research on the Changing Nature of the Brain

One of the most important recent discoveries regarding the brain is its neuroplasticity. Simply put, neuroplasticity means that our brains change with repeated experience. Also of importance is that emotion now appears to be central in the study of neuroplasticity. Furthermore, considerations regarding the importance of stress, anxiety, and emotion have become important avenues of research in the development of healthy psyches.

To underscore the importance of these considerations, the National Institute of Mental Health (NIMH) recognizes the intricate relationships between stress, anxiety, emotions, cognition, and brain biochemistry and has established several important areas for current and future development. Among these proposed areas of research are the effect of stress hormones on learning and memory, the role of emotion in cognition, and cognitive research in depression and anxiety disorders. Additionally, the NIMH has identified important areas of future research regarding the constantly changing nature of the human brain. These identified areas include generation of new nerve cells in the adult brain, the role of stress in nerve cell regeneration, and the plasticity of the human brain.[10]

The NIMH encourages this line of investigation because its scientists report constant changes in the functioning of the brain resulting from new memories, the addition of new neurons, changes in hormones, and stress and trauma. They regard this plasticity of the brain as an integration of nature versus nurture and conclude that it is through this plasticity that experience is constantly changing the brain.[11] Researchers once believed that the brain, once formed, could not produce new brain cells, but now the production of new adult nerve cells in the brain has been scientifically validated. Brain cell production and the strengthening of neural response appears to happen through repeated experience, and recent research has shown that stress and anxiety appear to decrease nerve cell regeneration in the brain.[12]

It has been shown that negative emotion plays a strong role in the stress response as well as memory formation and the development of anxiety. Changing the emotional response during stressful situations may profoundly affect the stress response, development of anxiety, memory formation, new brain cell generation, and overall cognition. Moreover, a depressive mental schema, a tendency to view the glass as half empty rather than half full, physiologically predisposes a person to the development of depression and may perpetuate the illness. Intervention tools to create emotional resilience through the experience of positive emotion may help improve the depressive mental schema.

If experience is constantly changing the brain, evoking positive experience and emotions through appropriate intervention techniques is a promising avenue for positive brain development.

Summary of Emotion Research

What all this research in the area of emotion has shown us is that there is powerful potential in the study of intentional cultivation of higher emotional feeling states that lead to living healthier, stronger, and more productive lives. There is potential in creating positive affect in our lives by feeling and operating from higher emotional states. There is potential in improving our cognition, changing our perceptions and judgments, reducing depression and anxiety, and creating different mood states through which we perceive and interpret our world. Most of all, there is potential in the generation of new brain cells and through the plasticity of the brain, creating new neural networks that function from higher emotional states.

The Importance of Feeling

When we begin to examine the physiological process of intentionally cultivating and routinely experiencing higher emotional states, it is important to remember that the experience of emotion involves much more of the brain than does conscious thought. Also, remember that the feeling aspect of emotion creates the biochemical shift in our bodies. The feeling aspect of emotion, not as a passive state responding to external stimuli but as purposeful intent, is paramount in our intentional cultivation of higher emotional states. The feeling state of these higher emotions comes from our internal selves.

Chapter One shared research by Alexander Astin. In his article "Why Spirituality Deserves a Central Placed in Liberal Education," Astin argues that the capabilities of the unconscious mind are nothing short of awesome. He states that this nonconscious part of the mind is the source of our intuition, inspiration, creativity, and spirituality, and these qualities come pretty close to what constitutes the aspects of mystical experiences.[13] In another article Astin and Keen attempt to describe what a highly developed spiritual person would "look" like. Through their research they identify a component called *equanimity*, which appears to capture some of the qualities associated with higher states of consciousness.

Equanimity, or the capacity to "see the silver lining" during difficult or trying times, appears to have a strong affective component. It is associated with terms like "felt at peace," "feeling good," and "felt a strong connection."[14] What these two articles contribute to our exploration is that intuitively we know that the nonconscious mind is the source of those qualities we associate with states of higher consciousness; these states carry a heavy "feeling component" to them. We feel intuition, we feel inspiration and creativity, we feel at peace, and we feel higher emotional states.

Again the field of positive psychology tells us that we don't have to be a passive vessel responding to external stimuli; instead, we need to be exploring ways to intentionally reach our higher potential. If it is our intention to reach a higher potential or higher states of consciousness, to develop a sense of equanimity, we need to explore ways to reach this nonconscious part of our mind. A conscious intent to create feeling states of higher emotion may be an effective way to do this. Throughout the rest of this chapter, we will examine the physiological process of why this works.

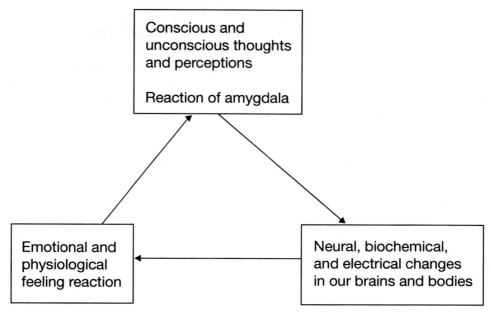

FIGURE 6.1   The circular nature of perception, physiology, and emotion

Turning the Tides

By now we should be acutely aware of the fact that where we keep our emotional attention or "feeling" attention every moment of every day profoundly affects who we are becoming. This process works whether we are conscious of it or not; it works whether we are using it to our advantage or not. In fact, most of this book so far has covered this process as we remain in status quo, when we behave as if we are at the mercy of all random external stimuli and as if it is our right to keep in negative mental states because circumstances have been bad to us.

Hopefully by now in this process we deeply understand that our perceptions, because of their biochemical, neural, and electrical impact on our bodies and brains, eventually become who we are. Furthermore, our biochemical, neural, and electrical patterns both affect and determine our perceptions. Such is the circular nature of perception, emotion, and attention. Because this pattern is circular and because it can result in a negative or positive spiral, at some point we need to be able to stop and reverse the process. It also is extremely important to remember that if even if a memory or perception is not conscious, it still can subconsciously influence our behavior, decisions, future perception, and health.

Figure 6.1 provides a visual interpretation of this circular process. Let's move on to examine scientific evidence of what happens when we can reverse this process. Redirecting our emotional attention to focus on higher emotional states changes our biochemistry, the neural patterns in our brains, and the electrical patterns in our hearts and throughout our bodies. In short, it changes us.

The goal of redirecting our emotional attention is to break this destructive cycle and replace it with a positive one based on the operation of higher emotional states. In the interpretative model represented in Figure 6.1, we originally perceive an event, either consciously or subconsciously, to carry some emotional impact for us. Once that perception has taken place in the amygdala, our bodies respond with corresponding biochemical, neural, and electrical impulses through our bodies. This is the physiological basis of emotion.

After this process has taken place, we begin to become aware and this reaction is brought to our attention through the recognition of the physiological feeling pulsing throughout our bodies, such as a racing heart, tightness in the chest, a wave of uneasiness, or the conscious processing of an emotional event. Remember conscious processing is when the whole process becomes subjective and is easily misinterpreted or misassigned unless you have acute understanding of what is really going on psychologically and physiologically throughout this process.

The impact of this event and its physiological and psychological ramifications then influence our perceptions. These events are happening so quickly they almost seem simultaneous; we feel a wave of physical and psychological responses, and our perceptions of the event begin to grow in severity.

Specific tasks and techniques to recognize and reverse this process are presented in the next chapter. In brief, this process involves recognizing, either by sensing our physiological reaction or by our conscious emotional attention, that we are having an emotional reaction, disengaging from that negative reaction, and making a conscious and intentional effort to redirect our emotional attention. These techniques can be used right in the moment of a negative emotional reaction as well as on a regular and consistent basis. Routinely doing this can change our physiological response patterns and the neural networks associated with our reactive patterns. In other words, we consciously and intentionally create positive higher emotional reaction experiences that ultimately replace the negative response patterns stored in the limbic areas and amygdala of our brains. In essence, we create a positive spiral, as represented in Figure 6.1, instead of a negative one.

The more we experience any emotional reactive pattern, the more that pattern becomes hardwired in our brains. These techniques are about consciously creating, by specific intent, positive reactive patterns as our normal mode of being. However, before these techniques are presented, it is important to have an understanding of the immense biochemical, neural, and electrical benefits resulting from higher emotional states. Again, all these psycho-physiological reaction patterns profoundly affect our perceptions and thus the circular nature of our emotional states. It is also important to underscore the point that this part of the brain provides meaning to our existence.

Biochemistry, Higher Emotions, and Oxytocin

Candace Pert, a leading research scientist in the molecules of emotion, argues that the idea that the brain is the only place we feel emotion is outdated and that our whole body really is our subconscious mind. She backs this point up with scientific evidence that the chemicals we associate with emotion can be found throughout the whole body, as evidenced by twenty-five years of mapping specific receptor sites associated with the biochemicals of emotion. What this all means is every time we have an emotional reaction, our body is flooded with chemicals representing that emotion.

These are usually in the form of peptides released throughout the body. Every cell in the body has receptor sites for specific peptides; and in essence, the peptides activate that cell. Additionally, each receptor site is specifically designated to receive only that peptide, or a similar class of peptides. Furthermore, these receptor sites may reside on surface membranes of specific organs and are responsible for activating the activity of that organ, including hormonal release.[15]

More simply, we have an emotional reaction and our body becomes flooded with chemicals specific to that emotion. Beyond the obvious activity in the brain, these chemicals are also sent throughout our whole body; they are sent to organs and other target cells and may cause additional hormonal reactions like the release of cortisol.

The bulk of these peptides is produced in the brain, with the limbic system serving as the main factory. What does this mean? When we have an emotional reaction, conscious or subconscious, an immense amount of peptides is produced and released from our brains. These peptides literally flood the body and control the activity of cells, organs, hormones, and other neurons. Every cell in the body has tens of thousands of receptor sites for specific peptides.[16] How we feel and act at any given moment is a result of the activity of these peptides and the biological process that ensues from their release. How we act, how we feel, any given moment of any given day is a result of these biochemical processes.

Relating back to our discussion of positive psychology and the idea that we as humans don't need to be regarded as an empty vessel only able to respond to external stimuli, the importance of these peptides should be obvious. By taking advantage of the ability to intentionally create states of higher emotional awareness and really feel those states, we can produce peptide reactions throughout our body that are conducive to further developing those states.

Another consideration, which will be discussed in more depth later in this chapter, is that the frontal cortex has been shown to strengthen and enlarge from routine focus on loving kindness as practiced in specific meditation practices. Much of our discussion of emotion has focused on the limbic system, but the frontal cortex is responsible for making choices, reasoning, and planning for the future. Pert suggests that as we move forward and upward in the brain from the limbic system to the frontal cortex, there are exponentially more opiate receptor sites.[17] Opiates are peptides associated with states of bliss. How she interprets these findings is that pleasure and bliss increasingly influence our criterion of choice. If we can create states of pleasure and bliss by intentionally focusing our attention on higher emotional states, we begin to make moment-to-moment choices for our attention and plans as a result of that blissful state.

The Power of Oxytocin

I believe one of the most promising avenues of recent research regarding the molecules of emotion and cultivating higher emotional states is in the area of the hormone oxytocin. Oxytocin has been historically referred to as the "bonding hormone" because of its release during breast-feeding and childbirth. Recently however, this hormone has been associated with numerous positive states, including trust, many types of bonding and closeness, and it has been shown to have a clear antianxiety effect. An examination of oxytocin is a perfect fit in our discussion of redirecting emotional attention from states of anxiety and fear to higher emotional states. Research by Uvnas-Moberg demonstrates that the calm and connection system as activated by oxytocin is in direct opposition to the fight or flight system as activated by cortisol and adrenalin.[18]

Oxytocin also has an indirect positive influence. It has been associated with the release of endorphins, which have been referred to as our body's own morphine, an opiate. If these chemicals act on parts of the brain associated with positive choices, attention, and planning, then it is conceivable that increasing our oxytocin levels actually makes us more capable of making positive choices. Remember, oxytocin is produced during activities associated with bonding, closeness, and caring behavior. When I presented this concept in one of my graduate classes, a student came up with the following equation:

Compassionate Thinking = Smarter Thinking

We can demonstrate how this is true down to the level of our physiology by revisiting the metaphor of the yellow kangaroo and the blue elephant. Say stress, anxiety, and negative emotional reaction patterns are the yellow kangaroo. Trying not to think of the yellow kangaroo just makes that image more persistent. The key is in replacing negative reaction patterns with those of higher emotional states, represented by the blue elephant. It's easier to replace the image of the yellow kangaroo with the blue elephant. In the same way, we can replace the destructive effects of the molecules and hormones of negative emotion with the molecules and hormones of positive, loving emotions. In the process we achieve our own higher potential, connect more, bond more, trust more, and live a much calmer and connected life.

Uvnas-Moberg, one of the world's premier researchers on oxytocin, calls it the hormone of calm, love, and healing. Several other researchers have shown the powerful effect of oxytocin on trust by demonstrating that higher levels of oxytocin create more thriving conditions in economics and business.[19] Oxytocin plays a key role in many positively associated situations and conditions that may appear on the surface to be very different but are defined by feelings of contentment, peace, relaxation, and emotional closeness.

Oxytocin works through nerve branches that link to important areas of control in the brain and through the bloodstream. The hormone is both influenced by and influences important neurotransmitters associated with positive mood like dopamine and serotonin. Most importantly for our discussion, according to physician and researcher Kerstin Uvnas Moberg, even thought, associations, and recalled memories can release oxytocin in the body.[20] In *The Oxytocin Factor*, Uvnas Moberg paints a convincing picture of the power of oxytocin in activating the system she terms "the calm and connection system." In our examination of oxytocin, which draws heavily on her work, we will look at some of the benefits of oxytocin, some external activities that influence its production, its relationship with the stress hormones cortisol and the amygdala, and possible activities that stimulate its production through conscious intent. We will also take a brief look at the importance of oxytocin in sexual bonding as it relates to healthy partner choices, a topic we will explore more in Chapter Ten.

The benefits of oxytocin are vast. Some might question whether one hormone could be responsible for so many positive effects, physically and psychologically. Because research on oxytocin is fairly new, those questions are not uncommon. However, two important points need to be addressed in response to that concern. First, oxytocin, because of its link to important control systems in the brain, fuels many chain reaction benefits throughout the body. Our body's biochemical responses, neural responses, and electrical responses are intricately related to the release of this hormone. Second, we know the tremendous negative effects initiated and stimulated by the production of cortisol. If we can accept that cortisol is a trigger responsible for a whole cascade of negative effects throughout the body and brain, why question the positive effects of oxytocin? Again, this may be evidence of our willingness to focus on and accept the negative much more easily than to consider the positive.

Oxytocin is correlated with lower blood pressure and lower levels of the stress hormone cortisol. Oxytocin has been associated with more sociable and nurturing contact. Rats injected with oxytocin preferred closer contact with other rats, and that contact stimulated the release of more oxytocin. They were also less fearful, more curious, and more likely to explore unfamiliar surroundings. Additionally, rats in the same cage as those injected with oxytocin, but not injected themselves, also exhibited calmer behavior. Thus, biochemically induced behavior appears to affect not only us, but those around us. Oxytocin has been associated with bonding attachment and positive social memory from stimulation of the amygdala. When oxytocin levels have been high in relationship with another through bonding or connection, that relationship is likely always to be special to us through the activation of social memory.[21]

Oxytocin has been shown to reduce pain, reduce anxiety, and increase learning in addition to producing feelings of well-being, calm, and quiet. This feeling of calm and quiet well-being appears to be associated with its cortisol-lowering effects. If you remember from our discussion of the origination of the stress response, ACTH in the hypothalamus is the main precursor to the release of cortisol. Through its effect on the entire stress control system, oxytocin appears to lead to the reduction of ACTH and ultimately lower levels of cortisol. As a result, oxytocin has a direct role in alleviating the negative physiological and psychological responses produced by cortisol throughout our bodies. Oxytocin counteracts these effects.

By now, we should be acutely aware of the negative effects of cortisol and the positive effects of oxytocin. The question then becomes how we increase our levels of oxytocin to gather all those benefits. Before we explore ways to produce oxytocin by conscious intent, we will look at other activities that produce oxytocin automatically. The original study of oxytocin was in regard to childbirth and its release as a woman nurses her baby. Oxytocin is also released in high amounts in both sexes during many types of sexual behavior, as in touching and kissing, as well as during orgasm, which releases a flood of the hormone into the bloodstream.[22]

Oxytocin has been shown to increase as a result of massage, connective conversations, a shared meal, meditation, and many types of bonding and trusting relationships. The hormone is produced in brain cells but also in reproductive organs, the gastrointestinal tract, the lungs, and the heart.[23] It is one of the reasons why we may feel content and happy after a meal or after sex and why taking several deep breaths helps to calm us down; it may be a contributing factor in why coherent electrical patterns of our heart make us feel better.

One root cause of the calming effect of these activities may be the activation of the amygdala, the storeroom of emotional reactive response, whether good or bad. Because of the production of oxytocin in vital organs and in the brain itself, it is important to examine the role of the vagal nerve in activating the amygdala. The vagal nerve is primarily responsible for bringing impulses from the body back to the brain.

According to Uvnas Moberg, these nerves probably go directly to the deeper parts of the brain, which deal with feelings and physiological reactions. Joseph LeDoux underscores this point by attributing impulses regarding the electrical activity of the heart to be transmitted directly to the amygdala. What is so significant about this process is that when the amygdala is stimulated with incoming information, it sends automatic responses by the way of feelings and physiological reactions throughout the body. When the amygdala is stimulated in a positive way, through a complex physiological process, we are flooded with feelings of calm, connection, security, love, and other higher emotional states.

One of the places oxytocin is produced is in the gastrointestinal system. This is why we feel calm or content after we eat and why some people who suffer from depression eat to ease psychological pain. Oxytocin also seems to be more responsive to foods higher in fat, which we often describe as "comfort foods." Because sharing a meal produces oxytocin, and the corresponding feelings of bonding and trust, it is often used as a positive way to conduct business. Additionally, the idea of the family meal actually has a physiological basis.[24]

Bonding with both humans and animals has been shown to increase oxytocin levels. Does just thinking about your dog or cat give you a feeling or rush of love or contentment? Does touching, holding, or being in close contact with your mate make you feel connected, calm, or content?

Let's return to the impact of oxytocin on endorphins. Uvnas Moberg suggests a strong connection between oxytocin and endorphins, the body's own internal opiates. In fact, oxytocin injections have been shown to increase the production of certain endorphins. Internal opiates are substances that are associated with producing a feeling of bliss or well-being.

We can connect this information to Pert's research showing that opiate receptors become denser as we move forward and upward from the limbic area of the brain into the frontal cortex. Again, the frontal lobe is the area of the brain associated with choice, planning, and reasoning. Working from this information it seems fair to conclude that practices to increase the production of oxytocin in our bodies and keeping our attention on feeling states of love, care, and compassion will create more positive choices, better and clearer reasoning, and planning based on optimistic outcomes.

The biochemical implications of our emotional states are profound. The impact of intentionally functioning from higher emotional states holds immeasurable promise. If we can intentionally create and function from higher emotional states and thus produce the circumstances that appear to be so beneficial from positive biochemical states, we have within us the power of transformation.

As we further our exploration of the promise and power of intentionally cultivating internal higher emotional states, we revisit the process of emotion in the brain. Remember the plasticity of the brain is in constant regeneration as a result of experience. Where we focus our current emotional and feeling state is perpetuated as continuing emotional states.

Imagine the power of intentionally shifting these states. If we can consistently shift our emotional and feeling attention to those states that stimulate positive reaction patterns from our amygdala, those positive patterns then cascade throughout our bodies. Imagine the possibilities for replacing experience and emotional memory. Imagine the possibilities for changing choice, for improving reasoning, and for planning from optimism.

Also, remember that repeated experience creates stronger and more efficient neural networks. If we intentionally and often shift to higher emotional states, we create the neural networks conducive to operating from those states more frequently. We replace negative emotional reaction patterns with higher emotional reaction patterns, stimulate subconscious and conscious neural and biochemical reactions throughout our bodies and brains, and change our perceptions.

The Heart's Electricity

Next we will examine the electrical patterns of our heart and how those patterns contribute tremendously to our internal states and external ways of functioning in the world. The heart is the most powerful generator of rhythmic patterns in the human body. Every time the heart beats, it sends an electrical impulse to stimulate its own contraction. This electrical impulse is what we measure when we take an electrocardiogram, or ECG. This electrical impulse is the strongest electrical impulse in the human body and we can gain a lot of information about the emotional state of the human body by studying the heart rate and pattern of impulse.

For instance, when we are stressed or anxious, our heart rate goes up, meaning the electrical impulse is activated more often. When we are relaxed, our pulse rate goes down. These electrical impulses are sent up the vagal nerve. These impulses travel straight to the amygdala, which releases information about our emotional state throughout the body.[25] If we keep in mind the importance of amygdala activation to the whole emotional state of the body, this point becomes very significant. Research has shown that electrical stimulation applied to the vagal nerve has increased electrical activity along this nerve tract and increased firing rates of neurons within both the amygdala and the hippocampus, and substantially influenced behavior.[26]

The amygdala and hippocampus both encode new experiences and activate stored emotional reactive response. In other words, these two parts of the brain sense the electrical patterns of our heart and release a whole set of emotional reactive responses based on those patterns of electrical stimulation. The amygdala can encode new experiences based on the activation patterns as well. As a result, consistently experiencing specific electrical patterns caused by intentional breathing will encode new emotional memory in the amygdala.

For instance, a measurement of heart rate variability—that is, the beat-to-beat changes in heart rate—has shown a very different sine wave pattern for breathing states associated with states of appreciation and those of frustration or anger.[27] What this means is that if the rate of the electrical impulse of the heart is plotted over time, it establishes a pattern that varies significantly depending on our emotional state. When we get frustrated or angry, we tend to take shallower, more inconsistent breaths than we do when we are calm or relaxed.

Additionally, when we intentionally breathe slowly, rhythmically, and deeply, this pattern establishes a smooth sine wave pattern. This pattern reflects the sympathetic nervous system being activated when we breathe in and the parasympathetic nervous system being activated when we breathe out. In other words when we breathe in, our heart speeds up, and when we breathe out, our heart slows down. If you know how to take your pulse, you can actually feel this process happening. The result, if we plotted the impulse as a time series pattern, would be a smooth and rhythmic up-and-down pattern.

Remember also, that another place oxytocin is produced is in the lungs. We will explore in Chapter Seven the many physiological changes that take place when we change the rate and depth of our breathing patterns. The changes in breathing patterns stimulate a cascade of positive emotional reactions throughout the body by the interaction of many different physiological systems. The emotional impact from all the stimulated changes from intentional deep breathing patterns is profound. Imagine these patterns as encoded electrical information being sent from the heart up through the vagal nerve straight into the amygdala. The amygdala senses this electrical information and either activates states of anxiety and fear from erratic shallow breathing or of calm, connection, or other higher emotional states from slow, deep breathing. These encoded patterns are responsible for firing neural networks associated with those emotional states.

The power here is that by intentionally shifting our emotional state to higher emotions and by breathing slowly, rhythmically, and deeply, we send an automatic impulse to our amygdala to release the neural impulses and biochemical state associated with that higher emotion. We also tell the amygdala to fire all the neural networks associated with that state. If we do it often enough, we encode a new, positive emotional memory deep in that reactive place in our brains. In other words, by intention and repetition, we begin to replace negative emotional reaction patterns and store higher emotional reactive patterns in that important part of the brain. By intention and repetition, we teach our bodies and brains to operate from higher emotional reactive states. By turning inward and intentionally changing our breathing patterns, we make it easier to cultivate higher emotional states based on love, kindness, care, compassion, and the like. We change the ways our bodies function, we change the way our brains function, and we change how we operate in the world.

A Conscious Intent to Feel Higher Emotions

I often hear comments like this: "How do I just choose to change my emotional state? I just can't not feel what I am feeling." I am not suggesting that you suppress emotion. Instead, I invite you to examine where those reactive states originate and to learn how to reset your own reactive neural networks and physiology to a higher emotional state so you can deal more coherently with the circumstances before you. Tools and techniques to achieve these states will be shared in the next chapter, but before we go on, it is important to share some research on what happens when people consistently and repetitively focus on higher emotional states.

You "feel" good, you "feel" happy, you "feel" at peace. You "feel" in the zone. You "feel" on top of the world, and you "feel" exhilarated. The amygdala provides meaning to your current circumstance in response to repeated experience. To train our feeling state, we need to activate our feeling state. Feeling and thinking are two different states, and there is a world of difference between thinking positively and feeling a higher emotional state. Chapter Seven explores this concept and its practical applications. Now we will explore evidence of how self-generated stimuli, rather than externally invoked stimuli, through thoughts and specific types of meditation can physically alter the brain.

In 2004, many leading neuroscientists from the West joined the Dalai Lama in India to examine the possibility of changing the structure and function of the human brain by conscious intent. The goal was to see if we could change the structure and function of the brain by intentionally controlling the way we think and feel and, conversely, change the way we think and feel as a result of changes in brain function. This meeting prompted a phenomenal amount of neuroscientific research, which yielded a wealth of important information regarding the plasticity of the human brain and possibilities of conscious intent.

Although our previous discussion regarding the origination of emotion focused primarily on the limbic system and more specifically the amygdala, the origination point was implicated as a result of external stimuli or unintentional activation through negative thought patterns. In other words, the emotional reactive patterns were exactly that—reactions to either external stimuli or to our own thoughts and feelings. One of the major findings of the research motivated by the meeting with the Dalai Lama was that the prefrontal cortex, the thinking part of the brain, could be intentionally used to activate a whole suite of emotions. More simply, we can intentionally use the prefrontal cortex and its strong connection to the feeling part of the brain to create emotional shifts.

This research led to the discovery that certain forms of mental training can transmit messages from the thinking part of the brain to the emotional part of the brain, eliciting more frequent and positive emotional responses.[28] Richard Davidson, one of the premier researchers in this area, found that even rudimentary forms of mental training could alter fundamental patterns of brain activity in those suffering from depression, and this training could actually induce plastic changes in the brain. He also asserts that more sustained training can shift the happiness set point and transform the emotional mind. This is accomplished by conscious activation of the left prefrontal cortex with the intention to create a higher emotional response.

What Davidson found was that certain types of intentional mental training could transform emotion and the brain circuits associated with emotion. More specifically, he found that certain types of meditation could strengthen the circuit leading to the limbic system and the activation of positive emotional states. In *Train Your Mind, Change Your Brain,* author Sharon Begley likens this process to a thermostat regulating the furnace of emotions; through this training we may be able to "rewrite the brain's emotional circuits, and forever alter our sense of well-being and contentment."[29]

Davidson found this evidence in his study of Buddhist monks. He postulated that this was evident in the monks because in the West we had no clue that mental training could change the brain's emotional circuitry; therefore, we never adopted the practices that would have shifted our baseline level of happiness in an enduring way.[30] In other words, all of us can reap these benefits, but the monks got there first by practicing this type of mental training. What is of extreme importance in this whole discussion and examination is that it is absolutely possible to change our baseline level of happiness and to transform our emotional mind, but that it takes intention, persistence, belief, and willingness.

These prerequisites will be examined as we further our journey. It is one thing to know about mental training for transformation and quite another to practice it. The routine experience of intentionally shifting emotional states promotes short-term and long-term change with all the resultant adaptations in our bodies, brains, and psyches. In the next chapter we begin to explore ways to move from "knowledge about" to "experience of." Lutz, Dunne, and Davidson clearly acknowledge that after reviewing the relative information regarding mental training, this collective evidence underscores the fact that "emotion regulation, including our very capacity for happiness and compassion, should be best conceptualized as trainable skills."[31]

No longer should we view emotion an inherent weakness, a hindrance to logical reasoning and cognitive functioning. Now we have the evidence to show that for the flip side of negative emotional reactive patterns, there is the hope, possibilities, and reality of intentionally cultivating higher emotional states by which to live. Research no longer focuses only on the negative aspects of emotion; it acknowledges that examining the positive aspects of psychology and emotion can lead us to higher potential. No longer is the brain viewed as a hardwired, unchangeable object; it is now viewed as a malleable organ that responds to external and internal experience.

Through the advent of positive psychology we are no longer viewed as empty vessels at the mercy of external stimuli. We can be in control of what fills our vessel. Through research examining individuals who have reached higher potential, we understand that they have been able to cultivate positive feeling states in which they truly feel at peace and connected. We understand that emotion is necessary for reason. The best cognitive function comes from a coherent emotional state. In fact, we have found that the amygdala provides meaning to context, and a person with a healthy emotional response system actually reasons much more effectively.

We now realize that the power lies in not just trying to reduce the negative, but in intentionally cultivating the positive. We understand that intentionally cultivating higher emotional states through connection, compassion, care, and loving kindness activates the emotion nodes specific to those states and cultivates more of the same. Where we keep our attention every moment of every day powerfully determines who we are becoming, whether we like it or not, whether those patterns are positive or not.

Through our knowledge of the emotional centers of the brain, we understand that because of the vast amount of emotional memory stored within these structures, we can only effectively process like emotional reactions at one time. If our attention is focused on anger, fear, jealousy, guilt, or any other negative emotional state, more of those like feeling reactions are stimulated, ultimately affecting our perception and ability to reason. Conversely, if our attention is focused on feelings of care, compassion, connection, or other higher emotional states, we can achieve higher reasoning, perceptions, and potential based on those states.

We now know that through the plasticity of the brain and intentional cultivation of nurturing external circumstances and internal development, we can change the functioning of existing neural networks. Additionally, we can create new neural networks, change the biochemistry in our bodies, and establish coherent electrical patterns in our hearts. Through connection, bonding, and consistent intentional cultivation of higher emotional states, we begin to replace the cortisol in our bodies with oxytocin and activate the "calm and connection system" rather than a flight or fight response.

Through the phenomenal research on the brain, we have learned that the frontal cortex, or thinking part of the brain, functions much more optimally when we practice to intentionally cultivate higher emotional states. Through consistent mental training, we can create profound changes in the structure and function of the brain, in the biochemistry of the body, and in the electrical patterns of the heart. Research has shown that the more one practices this mental training, the more significant the changes. For those who have put significant time into training on states of compassion, the connection between the frontal and emotional regions of the brain become stronger. In other words, mental training can alter connections between the thinking and the emotional parts of the brain, and we see clearer decisions as well as heightened empathy and love.[32]

We have learned that our whole body is affected by our emotional state, and we have the power to shift this state. We can no longer remain at status quo because now we know that status quo perpetuates more of the same. If we choose to focus, catastrophize, and ruminate or wallow in the negative, the negative is what is stimulated in our bodies and brains. Our higher potential is lost.

From this knowledge comes a crucial question: If we have all this information, the extreme possibilities for internal and external transformation, will we use it? If we now know that positive emotional patterns are an integral component for reason and decision making, will we take the necessary steps to begin the transformative process? We have the power to intentionally cultivate higher emotional states from which to live and, in doing so, profoundly change the way we operate in the world. But will we actually do it?

We have the information, and we have seen the possibilities. Now we need to examine our willingness to live from a more internally directed state of being. Are we willing to move beyond the status quo? Are we willing to intentionally and routinely cultivate higher emotional states through circumstance and internally redirecting emotional attention? Are we willing to reach our higher potential through looking inward? If we are not willing to do what it takes, why not? What is the payoff in staying stuck?

In our fast-food society, we are so accustomed to immediate results that we have lost sight of the value of sustained experience. Only through routine experience can we garner these changes, but routine experience takes attention and effort.

When I began examining these issues in my own life, I held the metaphor of a previously closed room. When the room was closed, I neither understood the potential nor the detriment of what was inside that room, and I lived my life in status quo. Once I opened the door, the door to my internal self, I found a room full of unlimited potential, but it was quite dusty and dirty from neglect. I knew that consistent intentional attention to my internal self and an inward focus on higher emotional states was all it would take to clean it, but I was not sure I wanted to put in the effort.

But now I had the knowledge, a clear understanding that not only was the room there, it desperately needed attention. Locking the door and walking away was not an option. In acknowledging existence of that room, I realized that I had vast potential in its existence. If I walked away, I remained stuck in the status quo, but the status quo was less bearable because I knew there were other unexplored possibilities.

From all the research on negative emotion, we know how destructive the status quo can be. To unlock the door to our higher potential, we need to be willing to take the first step, to look inward, to realize the potential of cultivating higher emotional states, and to make that potential our repeated experience. This repeated internal experience will reshape our brains, reshape the internal states of our bodies, reshape our relationships, and reshape our lives.

Now we begin to look at the transformative process in action. This is the focus of Part 2 of this book. In the next two chapters we will explore techniques aimed at intentionally cultivating higher emotional states. These techniques can help us reduce the stress and anxiety in our lives and achieve our higher potential. This is the most important information in the book. It takes the concepts we have learned regarding the importance and possibilities of creating higher internal experience and applies them concretely. Beginning in Chapter Nine, we entertain the question of willingness, and beginning with Chapter Ten, we will examine the transformative process through cultivation of external experience. Part 2 of this book presents concrete steps to create circumstances in our lives that are more conducive to creating and living from higher potential.

Higher Emotion Image List
EXERCISE AND REFLECTION #6

The key to transformation through neuroscience and the cultivation of higher emotional states is to change our physiological response patterns. By doing so, we change our brain's neural connections and biochemistry and, ultimately, our perceptions, behaviors, and way of being in the world. Creating a positive feeling response pattern requires us to genuinely feel a positive emotion or feeling state, not just cognitively think about it. It is the feeling state that activates the limbic system and produces the biochemical and neural cascade of positive emotional reaction patterns throughout the body.

This activity is the foundation of many to come and a key in training yourself to refocus your emotional attention.

Instructions: On the last activity you were asked to brainstorm and list what you experience as positive and negative emotions and roughly assign a height level to each as you placed it on the paper. Pick a few of the positive emotions or positive feeling states you listed in the previous exercise that especially resonate with you. Make a list of descriptions of people, places, things, actions, and thoughts that produce a genuine and sincere feeling state of these emotions. Whether it is gratitude, joy, loving kindness, compassion, peacefulness, love, serenity, or happiness, the key is to list and describe things that elicit these feeling states, what allows you to feel comfortable experiencing this feeling. It is important to describe situations that bring up only positive feelings states, not something that is initially positive but carries some degree of negative emotion. When I conduct workshops, I quite often characterize this as "love without the baggage," and that seems to make the point.

The key to this list is that it will be used as a tool to help refocus your emotional attention, so the things listed may not necessarily be the most important things in your life if those things are laced with challenge. Eventually you can train yourself to feel grateful about something in the challenging situation to separate that from the negative feelings associated with it, but this skill is usually cultivated after substantial practice. This list should include the simple as well as the complex.

For instance, for a quick, simple feeling of gratitude I focus on the feelings generated by my dog's face. She is ever-loyal and unconditionally loving. My children give me a much, much deeper sense of gratitude. The image of myself at the top of the half-dome in Yosemite or rafting down the Merced River in the warm sun generates a wonderful sense of peacefulness or serenity. All of these are appropriate for my list. Once again, the important point about the things you list are the feelings they generate. List and describe many. List and describe small things as well as big things. Brainstorm and be creative. After you have listed many images—real and imaginary—pick two or three and describe in depth the feelings they generate in you.

Higher Emotion Image List

_____

_____

_____

_____

_____

_____

_____

_____

_____

_____

_____

_____

_____

_____

_____

Reflect and Process

Describe in depth some of the things on your list, and, only focusing on the positive or higher emotional aspect, describe the feelings they generate in you.

_____

_____

_____

_____

_____

_____

_____

_____

_____

_____

_____

_____

_____

_____

REFERENCES

1. Csikszentmihalyi, M., *The Evolving Self* (New York: HarperCollins, 1993): 2.

2. Seligman, M. E. P. and M. Csikszentmihalyi, *"Positive Psychology: An Introduction,"* *The American Psychologist*, 2000, 55 (1), 5–8.

3. MacLeod, A., and R. Moore, "Positive Thinking Revisited: Positive Cognitions, Well-Being, and Mental Health," *Clinical Psychology and Psychotherapy* 7 (2000): 1–10.

4. Avia, M. D. "Personality and Positive Emotions," *European Journal of Personality* 11 (1), 33–56.

5. LeDoux, J., *The Emotional Brain: The Mysterious Underpinnings of Emotional Life* (London: Orion Books, 1998).

6. Joseph, R., ed. *Neurotheology: Brain, Science, Spirituality, Religious Experience* (San Jose, CA: University Press, 2003).

7. MacLeod and Moore, "Positive Thinking Revisited."

8. LeDoux, *The Emotional Brain.*

9. Gomez, R., "Neuroticism and Extroversion as Predictors of Negative and Positive Emotional Information Processing: Comparing Eysenck's, Gray's and Newman's Theories," *European Journal of Personality* 16 (2002): 333–350.

10. National Institute of Mental Health, *Cognitive Research at the National Institute of Mental Health* (Bethesda, MD: Author, 2000).

11. Ibid.

12. Brown, E. S., A. J. Rush, and B. S. McEwen, "Hippocampal Remodeling and Damage by Corticosteriods: Implications for Mood Disorders," *Neuropsychopharmacology* 21:4 (1999): 474–484.

13. Astin, A. W., "Why Spirituality Deserves a Central Place in Liberal Education," *Liberal Education*, 2004, 90 (2), 34–41.

14. Astin, A. W., and J. P. Keen, "Equanimity and Spirituality," *Religion and Education* 33:2 (2006): 1–8.

15. Pert, C., *Molecules of Emotion: The Science Behind Mind-Body Medicine* (New York: Scribner, 1997).

16. Ibid.

17. Pert, C., *Everything You Need to Know to Feel Go(o)d* (Carlsbad, CA: Hay House, 2006).

18. Uvnas Moberg, K., *The Oxytocin Factor: Tapping the Hormone of Love, Calm, and Healing* (Cambridge, MA: Perseus: 2003).

19. Zak, P. J., R. Kurzban, and W. T. Matzner, "Oxytocin Is Associated with Human Trustworthiness," *Hormones and Behavior* 48 (2005): 522–527.

20. Uvnas Moberg, *Oxytocin Factor.*

21. Ibid.

22. Ibid.

23. Ibid.

24. Ibid.

25. LeDoux, *The Emotional Brain.*

26. Miyashita, T., and C. L. Williams, "Glutametergic Transmission in the Nucleus of the Solitary Tract Modulates Memory through Influences on Amygdala Noradrenergic Systems," *Behavioral Neuroscience* 116:1 (2002): 13–21.

27. McCraty, R., and M. Atkinson, "The Effect of Emotions on Short-Term Heart Rate Variability Using Power Spectrum Analysis," *American Journal of Cardiology* 76:14 (1995): 1089–1093.

28. Begley, S., *Train Your Mind, Change Your Brain: How a New Science Reveals Our Extraordinary Potential to Transform Our Lives* (New York: Ballantine Books, 2007).

29. Ibid., 231.

30. Ibid.

31. Lutz, A., J. D. Dunne, and R. J. Davidson, *Meditation and the Neuroscience of Consciousness,* in Cambridge Handbook of Consciousness, eds. P. Zelazo, M. Moscovitch, and E. Thompson (Cambridge, Great Britain: Cambridge University Press, 2007): 87.

32. Begley, *Train Your Mind.*

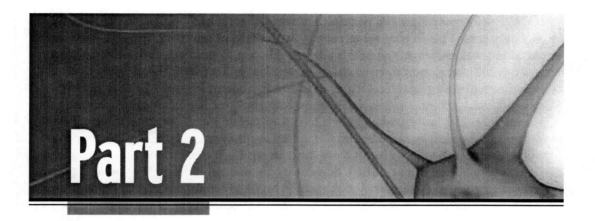

Transformation through Cultivated Internal and External Experience

The first part of this book has led us to the understanding that repeated experience basically creates our reality. Repeated experience creates stronger and more efficient neural networks in the brain, which influences perceptions and has a large impact on our behavior and choices. Repeated experience changes our biochemistry and makes our body more efficient at biochemically repeating those states. Repeated experience of breath control influences the electrical patterns emanating from our heart and directly transmitted to the amygdala, the brain's emotional processing center, which is in turn responsible for a whole host of psychological and physiological reactions throughout the body.

This process happens constantly and consistently, whether the experience is positive or negative and whether we are aware of it or not. It can empower positive spirals, expose us to negative spirals, or leave us at status quo. The most important point to grasp about this process is that it is repeated *internal* experience that creates these shifts. External circumstances certainly have an impact. Sometimes these circumstances can be horrific and seemingly impossible to overcome, but ultimately our internal processing of those circumstances, whether positive or negative, conscious or subconscious, determines our experience of those situations.

This is why two people can perceive and respond completely differently to the same set of circumstances. This is why some people, in the face of adversity, seem to have almost incomprehensible resilience, and others who would seem to have supportive external circumstances can still suffer from internal chaos, depression, and anxiety. This is why great wealth and advantage doesn't guarantee a happy or internally content life and why so many with vast wealth and fame commit suicide, suffer from drug abuse, or live internally chaotic and out-of-control lives. This is why, when people look for external success or external circumstances to fill the void they feel inside, they still feel empty inside even if they achieve that success.

Our internal experience creates these shifts in our bodies, brains, psyches, and lives, and our internal experience can be shifted. Sometimes the internal experience is the only place we can start. In my friend Alexander Astin's research on highly spiritually and emotionally developed people, he identified a character trait he defined as equanimity, or the ability to see a silver lining in every cloud, even in the face of adversity. It is my contention that this ability is a true and authentic internal experience of those people, and it is also my contention that this ability can be created and cultivated in each one of us. Intentionally cultivating positive, authentic, internal experience not only changes our bodies, brains, and behaviors, it can help us all to live up to a higher potential and live more productive and happy lives.

Our daily adversity may be the stresses, strains, or anxieties discussed in the first part of this book. Our daily adversity may be overcoming difficult emotional reactive patterns that were developed during difficult or challenging life experiences. Our daily adversity may be in battling our own internal chaos caused by stress, anxiety, or depression. Or, we may face the stress of external circumstances or time pressures, pressure to perform, or pressures in relationships. Our daily adversity may be in knowing that we could be living up to a higher potential, living a life in which we are thriving instead of just surviving.

How do we genuinely develop enough equanimity to live up to a higher potential, to live more productive and happy lives? How do we authentically create and cultivate our internal experience so it is more conducive to living lives free of so much internal chaos, stress, and anxiety? How do we authentically and genuinely see the silver lining as well as know that it is in that direction that we are headed?

Several dimensions of cultivating positive internal experience will be shared in this second part of the book. We will explore the intentional cultivation of higher emotional states through techniques designed to change our physiological reactions to the emotional unease caused by stress and anxiety and techniques designed to raise our baseline level of happiness. These practices are the most important information in this book; with consistent practice, they can transform how our bodies, brains, and psyches function. The power of consistently engaging in these types of practices can not be understated.

The second dimension we will examine is the practice of intentionally cultivating external circumstances so that they are more conducive to a positive internal experience. What aspects of our day-to-day lives either add to or detract from being able to spend more time in higher emotional states? Time makes experience, and the more total time we spend in higher emotional states, or internal coherence, the more that experience creates the neural and other physiological changes that can transform our way of being. In short, what are we exposing ourselves to on a daily basis? What does our "internal energy diet" look like?

With enough time and experience, we can raise our baseline level of functioning, or our baseline level of happiness as Davidson calls it.[1] This comes from intentional physiological practices and from intentionally creating conducive circumstances in our lives from which to grow.

The third dimension to intentionally cultivating positive internal experience is examining subjective interpretation of the external circumstance. A large part of this subjective interpretation will naturally begin to transform as our perception changes; however, we must maintain an awareness of how our interpretations powerfully affect our internal experience. In other words, how we see any situation powerfully affects our internal experience of that situation. Many times the emotional content of a situation is subject to interpretation, and that interpretation can powerfully influence the outcome. In other words, how we choose to see certain circumstances powerfully determines our physiological and psychological reaction, our perception, and ultimately the outcome.

A fourth dimension of creating transformation through internal experience is taking what you have learned about the physiological dynamics of internal experience and all the self knowledge you have gained throughout this process and putting it into action in your external lives. How do you now come back out of the labyrinth and live an external life of intention based on internal experience? How do you cultivate external circumstances that move you forward in the development of higher internal experience? This is similar to the second dimension proposed previously but at a higher level of intention.

In other words, the second dimension is at a more immediate level, such as recognizing people, places, things, or experiences in your daily existence that add to or detract from your emotional energy and taking action to elevate that experience. This fourth aspect is about identifying and taking major steps to cultivate external change. This step is about recognizing and honoring who you are internally, making a serious commitment to elevate your internal experience, cognizant of all the physiological and psychological implications, and creating external circumstances to support this change. My friend Michael would call this living more authentically, intentionally cultivating the external circumstances that we live by to promote a higher internal experience from which to grow.

The internal experience creates our reality. We can cultivate our internal experience by intentionally focusing on higher emotional states. We can improve our internal experience through turning inward. The internal experience of cultivated higher emotional states is the power within.

The first part of this book focused on all the physiological, psychological, behavioral, and perceptual aspects of internal experience, whether that experience is good or bad. It laid down the foundation of why intentionally cultivated higher emotional states change internal experience and our way of operating in the world. Now we will focus on the process of turning inward to intentionally cultivate higher states of internal experience with the knowledge that the internal experience creates the plasticity of change.

Specific topics are directed at these four general dimensions of internal experience. Topics primarily addressing internal change at our core include specific techniques to create physiological change and true willingness for change. These topics are covered in Chapters Seven through Nine. Next we address what I call "tilling the soil," or preparing for change. The topics of our energy diet, subjective interpretation (or the way we choose to see things), and the power of semantics in addressing internal experience or change at the day-to-day level are covered in Chapters Ten through Twelve. Finally, Chapter Thirteen addresses going forward to create the external circumstances in our own lives that allow us to live a more internally authentic and productive life full of intention.

Throughout this section are more focused journal exercises. As in the first part, these exercises are of fundamental importance because journaling enables us to more effectively access our internal processes and cultivate the experience of internal focus.

Repeated internal experience, based on all the scientific concepts previously presented, creates and strengthens neural networks in our brains, changes our biochemistry to those states more conducive to calm and connection, and changes the electrical patterns from our hearts to a more coherent state. All of these changes lead directly to the amygdala and our storeroom of either positive or negative emotional reactive patterns. Higher potential can be achieved by cultivating higher internal experience.

REFERENCE

1. Begley, S., *Train Your Mind, Change Your Brain: How a New Science Reveals Our Extraordinary Potential to Transform Our Lives* (New York: Ballantine Books, 2007).

CHAPTER seven

HEART Techniques for Change

Intention and Higher Emotion

The focus of this chapter is to present techniques for intentionally cultivating higher emotional states to produce physiological change. We have laid a firm foundation for the principle that our repeated internal experience shapes our neural networks, biochemistry, and electrical patterns of our heart. This internal experience can be a result of internal reaction to external circumstance or internal experience alone. Either way, our internal reactions, either conscious or subconscious, create the measurable changes in our physiology and brain patterns that eventually become the way we perceive and behave in the world.

What does this mean? It means that how we feel at any given moment powerfully determines our physiological reactions, which in turn affects our perceptions and behaviors. We may feel reactions as a result of circumstances, or we may feel reactions because we are accustomed to operating from a specific emotional state. Because conscious processing is subjective, there is immeasurable power in being able to inspire change from intentionally cultivating higher emotional reactive patterns from the physiological level. In other words, we address reactive patterns where they originate, replace them with higher reactive patterns, and respond to our world differently. That's the focus of this chapter. By intentionally cultivating higher emotional reactive patterns from the level of our cells in our brains and our bodies, we may live up to a higher potential.

This chapter describes how to begin the process of intentionally cultivating higher internal experience within the reality that is our lives. This process in no way reduces the importance of external experiences or suggests that suppressing or ignoring emotion is a healthy practice. Cultivating external circumstances—the aspects of our daily lives—so that they more positively contribute to our internal states is of utmost importance and will be examined at length in later chapters. Additionally, suggesting that cultivating positive internal states at the physiological level is a powerful tool for transformation in no way implies that negative emotions should be suppressed or ignored. But, by this point in our journey, it should be clear that where we keep our emotional attention much of the time is a choice, although if we are conditioned to a specific pattern of emotional reaction, we may not even be aware we have that choice.

For instance, I have two friends with completely different outlooks. One can walk into a room of people and see individuals with a wide variety of positive attributes. The other can walk into the same room and see a room full of dysfunctional people. Both could cite plenty of evidence to support their perspectives, but the person who naturally sees the positive attributes will pull out more of the same from the people she encounters, thus allowing herself a wholly different internal experience, complete with the cellular reactions of a more positive biochemistry and more positive emotional reaction from deep inside her brain.

This chapter and Chapter Eight present techniques to intentionally change our physiology by consciously focusing on higher emotional states. We know the extreme damage we are doing to ourselves when we operate from negative emotionally reactive or stressful states. We know that positive psychology tells us that we don't have to be an empty vessel only responding to negative external circumstance, or our perceptions of negative external circumstance. We know that for our many negative physiological reactive patterns, we also have an equal number of positive reactive patterns, and we can cultivate those positive reactive patterns to live up to a higher potential. Repeated internal experience creates the physiological and neural patterns by which we live.

Higher Emotion and Refocusing Techniques (HEART)

The following techniques are about intentionally creating positive internal experiences and repeating those experiences often enough that they become our inherent operating patterns, physiologically and psychologically. These techniques are designed to be done in the moment of a negative reactive pattern to reduce and eventually transform that pattern. With sustained practice, we can change our baseline level of functioning, as Davidson puts it.[1] These techniques are about breaking the circular nature of perception and negative physiological and emotional reaction patterns to replace those patterns with positive reactive patterns.

The essential aspect of these techniques is that experience changes us. These techniques need to become repeated to be effective. The word *transformation* captures the process of change, with *trans* meaning "moving" and *form* referring to our current state. Wayne Dyer breaks down the word *transformation* as using action to move beyond our current form.[2] Transformation won't happen without action.

Experience is the necessary component of elevating our psychophysiology to positive or higher reactive states, as opposed to those states that harm us, keep us in status quo, or keep us filled with stress and anxiety. These techniques are much like exercise, in that you have to actively and routinely engage in doing them to reap their benefits. Like many things in life, you can't just read about them or think about doing them. You must experience them again and again. It bears repeating: Repeated experience is what changes our brains. If the experience component is missing, change will not become manifest.

As each aspect of the techniques is presented, the physiological foundation will also be shared to underscore the scientific basis of being able to cultivate an emotional shift. Along with the techniques, you will find several activities to process and complete to better prepare you to effectively practice the techniques. Finally, suggestions and activity/reflection exercises directed at cultivating routine practice will be presented to help you make the voyage from knowledge to experience, always with the idea that repeated experience produces change.

The techniques are presented in a basic format so they are easy to remember and implement. They are designed to work with our physiological processes to induce higher functioning states by bringing our feeling attention to higher emotional states. These higher emotional states induce our brains, our biochemistry, and the electrical patterns in our hearts to function from greater clarity, coherence, connection, and compassion and to change our perceptions and behaviors. These techniques are about intentionally cultivating higher emotional feeling states to purposely shift our psychophysiology to greater productivity, higher potential, and more positive internal and external experience. They are designed to work from the inside out, as the internal process ultimately creates the external experience.

The techniques are based on three basic steps and are designed to be modified depending on the circumstance in which they are used. The goal of these Higher Emotion and Refocusing Techniques (HEART) is to make the science of transformation accessible. These techniques are based on the wonderful information we have garnered through research of the stress process, emotion, and mental training. It is the "use of," not the "knowledge about," that produces change. My goal is to apply the gift of this information into a usable format.

HEART Basics

The simple steps of these techniques are:

Notice

Refocus

Choose _____

These steps are intentionally simple so you can keep them in mind, practice them regularly, and remind yourself that where you keep your emotional attention every moment of every day powerfully determines what is going on inside you. Even though the steps are simple, the physiological and psychological impact of routinely practicing them is profound. Let's explore the rationale and background for each step, as well as specific practices that need to be incorporated into each step to fulfill its purpose. Chapter Eight introduces the practical application, physiological background, and specific practices that need to be employed for HEART to succeed.

Notice

This step is most similar to the process referred to as "become the observer" or "cultivate the witness." This step is about training yourself to become acutely aware when you are having a negative, emotionally reactive, or stressful response to something and then disengaging from that response. Remember, the perpetrating event can be purely a thought or a feeling, not associated to an external circumstance. It can be anything that initiated this feeling. It may be a reaction to an external circumstance, person, event, or feeling, or it may be the feeling of emotional unease we associate with stress or anxiety.

It is also important to remember that this reaction may not necessarily be in your awareness. In fact, one of the major goals of this step is to train yourself to be aware when your body begins to shift to a negative state. Remember when we have a negative stressful or emotional reaction, one criterion that defines this reaction is that we have physiological reactions; simply put, the body responds. The activities on the feeling states of emotion and the identification of trigger points were designed to to direct your attention to how your body responds when you have either a negative stressful or emotional reaction.

Some people report a tightness in the chest, and some report that their heart pounds, they can't breathe, their stomach hurts, or they get a feeling of dread. Others notice the reaction in a psychological sense, as a feeling of fear or guilt or a sense of being overwhelmed. Many people experience both psychological and physiological responses. Everyone experiences this state differently, so you must learn to recognize your own reactions as they happen. One of my sons has learned to identify his typical set of reactions as "that feeling." He has trained himself to recognize and identify his reaction before he cognitively begins to process what is happening to him. "Mom, I am getting *that feeling* again," he tells me.

The most important aspect of this step is to learn to tune into how you are feeling physically and psychologically, as a reaction to something, which may be either internal or external. What usually happens is we have a physical reaction of which we may or may not be aware. Then, we have an emotional or psychological reaction, and we try to validate that reaction by whatever is in front of us at that moment, whether or not there is a connection between our response and the situation. Even if the situation warrants an emotional reaction, most often the magnitude of the reaction is out of context. If we can react in a calm, clear-headed way, we are much more able to produce coherent positive results. We don't have to succumb to negative emotionally reactive patterns to get things done.

Years ago, I was at Yosemite with two girlfriends. We had decided on a whim to hike up to Half-Dome, and we certainly didn't look the same as the prepared hikers going up the mountain that day. However, what wasn't apparent to others is that we were in good shape and certainly capable of completing the sixteen-mile hike. We ran into an arrogant male on the trail who asked us where were heading. I told him Half-Dome, and he made it very clear that he thought we were vastly overestimating our hiking ability. My friends always tease me because as they stood behind me, they could see my arms tense up and my fists become tight, and I wasn't even remotely aware that I was having that physical response. However, I did become aware that I was very angry that he could have been so arrogant as to stop us and treat us that way, and the whole rest of the day I carried that anger.

This is just a simple example of how this process may work. Ever since I was a young girl, I have had very strong reactions to any boy who told me I couldn't do something. Chances are the man who stopped us on the trail that day was not nearly as arrogant as I perceived him to be. Even if he was, I certainly didn't need to succumb to my reaction. I could have laughed it off and gone on with my day. But, in my mind, that man had really insulted us, and I carried that biochemical and brain reaction pattern throughout that day to prove it. In reality, I hurt myself by my reaction, not him.

To notice these reactions is to train yourself to become acutely aware of your own reactive patterns and to be able to identify them the moment they happen. My experience at Yosemite was a minor example of how this process works. My more serious reactive patterns usually involve a tightening of my chest, shortness of breath, sometimes a slightly nauseous feeling in my solar plexus (the area below the heart), and a general feeling of threat. Many times I feel general weakness, pressure around my eyes, and a general feeling of being overwhelmed. My goal is to recognize these physical reactions as soon as they begin and to stop myself from subjectively assigning them to the current situation and getting caught up in an emotionally reactive response. If I can disengage from the reactive response, I can more easily decide on a clear and appropriate reaction and proceed from there.

What are your reactive patterns? Where in your body do you most likely feel your response? It is important to remember that if you can feel the physical or psychological reaction, the process that has been the subject of most of this book has already begun. Your biochemistry has already been affected; your amygdala has surely already activated a whole host of physiological changes throughout your body, brain, and heart.

The second component of the notice step is to be able to disengage from the reactive pattern you are experiencing. This is the where the terms "cultivate the witness" or "become the observer" seem appropriate. Both of these terms convey the idea of disengaging enough from whatever reactive pattern you are feeling to be able to objectively observe that pattern. Keep this crucial point in mind: If you physically and/or psychologically feel the reactive pattern, the physiological process we have been examining has already begun; now you need to do what you can to disengage from and reverse that process.

Refocus

The refocus step involves refocusing your physical attention. Beginning to refocus your physical attention automatically activates the parasympathetic branch of your autonomic nervous system. In other words, by doing certain techniques, you can train your body to automatically calm itself down. We have what is called an automatic relaxation response built into our nervous system, and we can take specific steps to physically invoke this response.

The first step under Refocus is to pay attention to and intentionally relax the muscles and tightness around your eyes. The eyes are strongly connected to the limbic system. They powerfully reflect what is going on for us emotionally—thus, the sayings "the eyes are the window to the soul" or "look in his eyes to see if he's lying." You can fake a smile with your mouth, but you can't fake a smile with your eyes.

However, eyes and emotion are a two-way street. If you can pay attention to and relax and release all the tension surrounding your eyes, you send a powerful message to your limbic system to calm your whole emotional response system. The second step under Refocus is to release the tension in your shoulders. The shoulders are also subconsciously activated with stress, and releasing tension there helps your whole system relax. The third step is to bring your attention to a comfortable spot in your chest. I like to think of a ladder, stepping down from the eyes to the shoulders to the chest.

Several things happen physiologically when you bring your attention to the area of your chest, but first you need to decide where it feels comfortable for you to bring that attention. Many traditions use the heart, or the area around the heart, as the spiritual center of the body. Some Christian religious traditions refer to the "sacred heart," while some Hindu, Bon, and Buddhist traditions involve the heart chakra or the assemblage point. Quakers and Muslims also have specific reference to the heart and the solar plexus is generally believed to be an energy center right under the heart. If you ask people to place their hand on the part of their body where "they" are, most people place their hand on their heart or in the middle of their chest.

Some people are uncomfortable with references to the heart because of past painful or negative emotional reactive patterns associated with love. In this case, the solar plexus or the area around the heart is a good place to focus your attention. The solar plexus is considered one of primary energy centers of the body, and physically we know the heart plays a central role in the nervous system. Use whatever terminology you prefer and bring your attention to wherever it is physically comfortable for you to do so.

A crucial aspect of bringing your attention to that area of the chest is where your attention isn't. In other words, when we bring our attention to our chest, it isn't on our racing thoughts. There is a spot on the left temporal lobe that is responsible for the constant chatter that seems to repeat in our head all day every day. This constant chatter, when it is reacting to negative emotional states, exacerbates and exaggerates those states by perpetuating the negative emotional cycle described earlier in this book. When we are stressed, that chatter explodes, which then creates more stress.

The chatter from the cortex of the brain sends information to the amygdala, which then reacts with emotional reactive patterns, which in turn exacerbate the chatter. Information is constantly sent back and forth between these centers of the brain, and intentionally and effectively bringing our attention to our heart or a comfortable area in our chest quiets this process. If we don't take steps to quiet this process, our bodies and brains succumb to the full force of a negative emotional or stress reactive pattern. The simple process of bringing our attention to a comfortable or sacred spot in the chest helps to disengage from this negative process.

The last part of the Refocus step is to breathe. Breathing slowly, deeply, and comfortably activates several physiological systems that help slow down or reverse the stress, anxiety, or negative emotional reactive processes. This kind of breathing activates the parasympathetic nervous system and the automatic relaxation response in our bodies. In other words, our bodies automatically calm down physiologically when we breathe slowly and deeply.

In addition to invoking the relaxation response, our bodies appear to create more oxytocin as a result of deep slow breathing. One of the places in the body that oxytocin is produced is in the lungs, and this type of breathing appears to increase its production. Also, remember that increased levels of oxytocin not only activate the calm and connection system, they block the activity of cortisol in the brain. Our bodies change biochemically when we breathe slowly, deeply, and comfortably.

In addition to the automatic relaxation response and oxytocin production, Pert identifies a well-documented link between peptides and the respiratory tract. She states that nearly every peptide in the body can be found in the respiratory center and that changing the rate and depth of our breathing changes the quality and type of peptides released from the brain stem.[3] Again, consciously controlled breath patterns have a powerful effect on our biochemistry.

Finally, when we breathe slowly, deeply, and comfortably, the electrical patterns of our heart create a smooth sine wave pattern. Heart rate variability is a measure of beat-to-beat changes in heart rate. When plotted over time, the pattern that this plotting creates can be very distinctive. When we breathe slowly and deeply, this pattern creates a smooth and even sine wave.

According to Joseph LeDoux, electrical patterns from our heart are transmitted directly to the amygdala, giving important information to the primary emotional center in our brain regarding our state of calm. Keep in mind that the amygdala processes and perpetuates like information. That is, the information relayed to the amygdala regarding the state of excitement of the heart will stimulate the amygdala to release emotional reactive patterns consistent with the information it receives from the heart.[4] If our amygdala receives the electrical information as being calm and coherent, it will stimulate emotional reactions consistent with those states. However, if it receives the electrical information as being chaotic and out of sync, it will respond to those states.

Breathing slowly, deeply, consistently, and comfortably creates smooth coherent electrical patterns emanating from our hearts and fed directly to the emotional control center in the brain. This type of breathing appears to have a direct influence on our biochemistry by the oxytocin produced in the lungs and the other peptides produced by the respiratory control system. A final benefit is that this type of breathing has a direct impact on the automatic relaxation response invoked by the parasympathetic nervous system.

Choose _____

The last step in the HEART technique is to intentionally cultivate a feeling of a higher emotional state. I call this choose _____ because which higher emotion you focus on will vary based on the situation and timing. Additionally, genuinely making a feeling shift is the primary component, and it needs to be a sincerely felt emotion. Here is where we make the transition that positive psychology is beginning to address. Instead of only trying to reduce the negative, as traditional stress management techniques have suggested, we make an intentional effort to cultivate those emotional states that produce the physiological and biochemical shifts identified in Chapter Six.

In other words, we make an intentional effort to cultivate emotional states that will facilitate the production of oxytocin and reduce the impact of cortisol. We make an intentional effort to cultivate emotional states that access a positive emotional response from the amygdala, complete with the cascade of physiological effects that reaction will incur. We make an intentional effort to completely change our physiological and neural response patterns. Continually doing so creates the repeated experience needed to establish these as our new automatic response patterns.

How does all of this work physiologically and psychologically? The specifics of how to perform each step will follow shortly; however, the idea behind the Choose _____ step is that after we disengage from the negative emotional reaction we are experiencing, we intentionally cultivate a different reactive pattern. We do this by shifting our attention to a higher emotional state. Before examining the specifics of how and when to do this, let's first examine the physiological and psychological aspects behind this step.

From all the research shared thus far, we know that experience can induce changes in brain regions involved in regulating emotion. These changes are most likely due to the changes in the structure and function of the neural networks governing emotion. We also know that our internal processing, which is largely subconscious, activates the systemwide cascade of bodily reactions when we feel an emotional reaction. Furthermore, we know that our conscious thought process, in the form of thought, attention, or explicit memory, can have a profound effect on the activation of our emotion neural networks.

Intentionally placing our thoughts or attention on higher emotional states, and vividly trying to feel the effects of those states, creates new experience. Because of the strong connection between the thinking part of the brain and the feeling part of the brain we can intentionally shift the attention of the thinking part of the brain to higher emotional states, and transform our emotional reactive mind. The more we can effectively do this, the more these types of experiences are created and the more our neural circuitry is influenced. As Davidson said, "We can think of emotions, moods, and states of compassion as trainable mental skills."[5]

In his book *Synaptic Self*, LeDoux makes a big distinction between explicit memory and implicit memory. *Explicit memory* refers to memories we can consciously recall, while *implicit memory* is in more control of our inner life, reflected more in the things we do and the way we do them.[6] However, once more, because of the strong connections between the thinking part of the brain and the emotional part of the brain, we can intentionally recall explicit memories to induce implicit memories. To put it more simply, we can intentionally recall something that has significant meaning for us in our conscious mind to induce all the positive physiological reactions stored in our subconscious that influence our bodies and our brains. In other words, we can purposely recall, and intentionally feel, something that carries significance for us and induce a positive reaction throughout our body.

When I vividly recall, and let myself feel, a significantly positive emotional memory or connection to something, my body and brain responds to that experience with a positive reaction. That reaction in turn changes my perception and possibly my behavior. I am creating my own internal experience. When I routinely do this, I not only bring about immediate changes in my brain, body, and perceptions, but I also begin to establish long-term reaction patterns that are strengthened by repeated experience. I begin to use my ingrained emotional reactive patterns to my advantage.

Recall the mood congruency hypothesis, which tells us that because we have enormous amounts of emotional or reactive memory stored in the subconscious parts of the brain, we can only process like reactive patterns at a time. In other words, if I'm feeling happy or full of loving kindness, and that is where my attention is focused, I will create more of the same perceptions. Unfortunately, this is also true if I'm feeling angry, frustrated, overwhelmed, or immersed in another negative reactive pattern. Perceptions based on these reactive patterns then influence our behavior, the way we think and the way we act.

We can, however, use the mood congruency hypothesis to our advantage. Because we are conscious beings, we can control whether what Antonio Damasio calls the "would be inducer image" is allowed to remain a target of our thoughts.[7] We can control, in part, the nonconscious triggering of emotion through intentional conscious thought. If we have what LeDoux calls a "mood congruity of memories,"[8] and we can control what explicit memories, connections, attachments, or simply made-up positive feelings we choose to focus our consciousness on, we can influence our nonconscious emotional reactive patterns and create new experience. In other words, by choosing to focus on and feel higher emotional states, we create higher emotional response patterns. Additionally, the more we do this, the more those higher reaction patterns become ingrained response patterns. Repeated experience creates and strengthens synapse patterns and neural networks. As LeDoux says, "You are your synapses."[9]

In this chapter I have presented easy formulaic steps and the corresponding background physiology to begin to refocus our emotional attention to live less negatively reactive lives. Routine experience of these steps will transform your physiology, your reactive patterns, and your way of interacting in the world. There is incredible power from intentionally cultivating higher emotional states. In the next chapter, we will examine how these techniques can and should be incorporated in everyday life.

REFERENCES

1. Begley, S., *Train Your Mind, Change Your Brain: How a New Science Reveals Our Extraordinary Potential to Transform Our Lives* (New York: Ballantine Books, 2007).

2. Dyer, W., *The Power of Intention: Learning to Co-Create Your World Your Way* (Carlsbad, CA: Hay House, 2004).

3. Pert, C., *Molecules of Emotion: The Science behind Mind-Body Medicine* (New York: Scribner, 1997).

4. LeDoux, J., *The Emotional Brain: The Mysterious Underpinnings of Emotional Life* (London: Orion Books, 1998).

5. Begley, *Train Your Mind*, 221.

6. LeDoux, J., *Synaptic Self: How Our Brains Become Who We Are* (New York: Penguin, 2002).

7. Damasio, A., *The Feeling of What Happens: Body and Emotions in the Making of Consciousness* (San Diego, CA: Harcourt, 1999).

8. LeDoux, *Emotional Brain*, 212.

9. LeDoux, *Synaptic Self*, ix.

CHAPTER eight

HEART in Action

The Importance of Routine Experience

Although the physiological background of the HEART steps are extremely important in understanding the significance of refocusing our emotional attention, the routine and practical experience are essential. How do we begin to use these physiological and psychological concepts to our benefit? How do we create our routine experience of these concepts in sufficient enough magnitude to facilitate change? How do we practically use this information in our everyday life?

The power behind these concepts is built on new scientific knowledge of ancient wisdom practices. These techniques are certainly not the only answer to creating internal change through sustained mental practice, but they are easy to use and based on scientific principles and research focusing on sustained mental practices that have shown phenomenal positive changes in the human brain, body, and psyche. They were developed because of my deep belief that keeping our attention on higher emotional states profoundly affects who we are and how we function in the world.

HEART is purposely simple. Unless we can engage in the experience that creates change on a routine and consistent basis, it will remain "knowledge about" rather than "experience of." These techniques are simple so they can be remembered and practiced. They are simple so they can be done anytime, anywhere. They are represented and repeated several times throughout this chapter, in several formats, to optimize absorption. The more you can internalize, remember, and practice, the more effective HEART will be.

These techniques were created so they can be done in the middle of a reactive pattern and so that they can be done anytime we feel a higher physiological functioning will help us reach a higher potential. They were created for sustained practice to raise our baseline level of emotional functioning. They will be broken down into two models of practice, one to be done in the moment of stress, or whenever a higher level of emotional functioning in the moment will beneficial, and one for sustained practice for longer and more routine experience. Remember, consistent and routine experience creates change. I can't impress enough that our brain responds to and adapts to the experiences we routinely give it. There is power in intentionally cultivating higher emotion. There is more power in routinely experiencing these states. We begin this chapter by exploring the steps and substeps of these techniques. Specifics of how and when to perform the techniques will follow.

Each step should be done slowly and deliberately with conscious intent. Although the steps seem simple, there is an incredible amount of physiological change inherent within each step.

HEART in the Moment

Notice

Notice your physical reaction.

Notice your psychological reaction.

Disengage from any emotionally reactive response and physical reaction you are having.

Refocus

Release your eyes.

Release your shoulders.

Tune your attention to your chest, heart, assemblage point, solar plexus, or wherever feels comfortable for you.

Breathe slowly and deeply, but most of all comfortably (keeping your shoulders and eyes relaxed as you do so).

Choose _____

Make an intentional shift to a higher emotional feeling state.

(Use the activities presented later in this chapter to help facilitate that shift.)

Intentional Cultivation

When making an intentional shift to a higher emotional feeling state, it is important to remember that we are using the conscious or cognitive part of our brain to induce reactions in the nonconscious part of the brain, as well as in our biochemistry and electrical patterns of our heart. The reason why this is important to remember is that we need to do what is effective for each one of us in the intentional use of the conscious part of the brain. In other words, this is very different from positive thinking because our intent is to reach the positive reactive mechanisms in the brain and body. More simply, we need to *feel* the reaction, not just think about it, and what is appropriate and effective for one person may be different than what is appropriate and effective for another.

Everyone is different in how they most effectively can intentionally cultivate a higher emotional feeling state, and when I suggest this strategy, it is still hard for most to move from the paradigm that we must be controlled by our circumstances or negative thought or emotional reactive patterns. Initially, most people I work with find it easiest to hold an image that for them induces that feeling state. For instance, if I am in a situation where I notice I am having a negative physical and physiological reaction to something, after I disengage from that reaction, refocus my physical attention, and breathe, I may consciously hold an image of my children. Usually when I think of my children, I feel a deep sense of gratitude that they are in my life.

If you choose to hold an image to help create the feeling state, it must be one that actually induces a positive or higher emotional feeling state. The feeling reaction associated with physiological and psychological shifts is highly individual. You must hold an image that induces a higher emotional feeling state for you. It must be an image that isn't clouded with negative emotions. Remember it is the intentionally cultivated feeling state that is important, not specifically the image. I sometimes refer to this as "love without the baggage." The image is just a tool for you to facilitate the intentional shift to consciously feel a higher emotion.

After a substantial amount of practice and experience making this internal shift, your body and psyche naturally want to respond this way. In other words, the automatic reaction becomes one of rebalancing and naturally gravitating to a higher emotional reaction, and the image is no longer important. At this point if you understand that gratitude, understanding, or compassion will rebalance you and completely refocus your internal and external experience to a higher potential for that circumstance, you can put your attention on that feeling and induce a positive reaction. Sometimes just identifying the desired feeling by the word will help induce that feeling state. What does the word *gratitude* feel like? Or *compassion*? Or *understanding*?

These are just three examples of word descriptions for higher emotional feeling states. There are obviously many, many more, and the ones that will be most effective for you are those that resonate the most with you. Look inward and get in touch with what you intuitively feel would be the highest emotional reaction you can shift to in that moment. Repeat that word and feel its essence, or "bathe" yourself in that feeling state.

Practices for Success

Different circumstances and different situations will determine different possible reactions. In other words, if you are in a highly upsetting, stressful, or negative emotional circumstance, it will probably be hard to shift to a high feeling of compassion. What works for me at this point is to shift to the feeling of unconditional love my dog has for me. When I hold an image of her face, I can usually shift to a feeling of gratitude for the love she has for me and really feel that appreciation. Remember, the best way to take care of yourself is to be in control of your own internal reactions, not from a place of denial or suppression but from a place of love, acceptance, and gratitude. Then, from that higher emotional state, you can make clear, coherent, and positive choices rather than negative and emotionally reactive ones.

At the end of Chapter Five you were asked to brainstorm and write what you perceive as positive emotional reactions or higher emotional states above a midline on the paper and negative reactions below the line. Refer back to that activity and add any higher emotional states you may have overlooked. At the end of Chapter Six you were asked to brainstorm and write about various people, places, experiences, animals, thoughts, etc., that would elicit some of those higher emotional states for you. The important thing to remember here is that the images are just tools to elicit that feeling state. Your goal is to intentionally cultivate a higher emotional feeling state, and all the accompanying positive physiological reactive patterns, by consciously directing your attention. It is also important to remember that these are just techniques I have created to help direct your attention; by their very nature, these techniques will change and evolve.

Look back over the activities in Chapters Five and Six. Review what for you feels like higher emotional states. Review the images you have described that may elicit those feelings for you. If you need to add, delete, change, or modify at this point, do so. Also if it is appropriate for you, imagine how you would train yourself to cultivate the feeling state of the emotion you listed, with or without an image. In other words, try to feel what that emotion "feels like" for you.

Since these techniques are personal, let me share an example of how I use HEART. Imagine that I am in a heated conflict with a coworker. I know it is in my best interest to behave from a clear-headed and emotionally coherent state, but I notice I'm beginning to get upset and anxious. I notice and tune into my physical reactions in my body. I notice that my chest has tightened, my breathing has become much shallower, and I have a knot in my stomach and a general sense of threat. I make a conscious decision to disengage; I "cultivate the witness" and "become the observer." I refocus my physical attention from that reactive pattern right in that moment by relaxing the tension around my eyes, relaxing my shoulders, bringing my conscious attention to a place that feels comfortable in my chest area, and I begin to breathe slowly, deeply, and comfortably.

I now begin to notice my body and mind calming down, and I make a conscious effort to intentionally focus my psychological attention on a higher emotional feeling state. From my brainstorming on the positive and negative emotional diagram, I recall that the feeling of gratitude, peacefulness, or loving kindness is an important state for my higher functioning, and I choose to intentionally cultivate one of those feelings. I remember that on my list of descriptions of things that induce positive feeling states, I listed rafting down the quiet and still river in Yosemite as one of the most profound feelings of peacefulness I have ever experienced.

I continue to keep my eyes and shoulders relaxed and my attention in my chest area, and I keep breathing deeply and comfortably. I now hold the image of myself on the raft in the sun, on the peaceful river floating among the beauty of the Yosemite valley, including Half Dome and El Capitan. Just the image of really letting myself feel that memory invokes a whole body response of relaxation, peacefulness, and clear and coherent thinking. My neural patterns in my brain change; because of the profound effect the changes in my breathing patterns elicit, my whole body begins to relax, and the intentionally induced feeling state creates profound biochemical shifts in my body. Imagine all of this has happened in less than a minute while I am still in the same place and same discussion, but I am fundamentally different in my body, my brain, my behavior, and the way I respond.

Now imagine being able to make this shift when you are in the middle of a difficulty with a loved one. Imagine being able to make the shift when you are nervous because of a job interview or a speech. How about when you are in traffic? Or a car accident? Or with too much to do and too little time to do it?

The situations will always vary and the benefits will increase exponentially the more you make a conscious effort to cultivate this type of internal experience. Additionally, it is also extremely important to remember that refocusing your emotional attention is effective not only under stressful or anxious conditions, but also at times when you just want to perform or behave at your best; when you want to achieve your higher potential. Throughout much of my doctoral work, as well as in writing this book, I have used these techniques to focus my emotional attention, think as clearly and coherently as possible, and perform my best.

I have said many times, and I will continue to repeat, that the repeated experience of anything creates and strengthens our neural networks and biochemical reaction patterns. These techniques are no different. To gain the physiological and psychological benefits these techniques have to offer, they must be practiced routinely and often. Not only will they create positive reactive patterns, they will help break the cycle of negative and destructive reactive patterns. However, they must be experienced. Experience produces change, not just the knowledge of how these techniques work.

Identifying Situations, Higher Emotions, and Images
EXERCISE AND REFLECTION #7

The more you can remind yourself to use these techniques in the moments they will be effective, the better off you will be. If you become negatively reactive in a situation and the reaction gets out of control, but you don't think about refocusing your emotional attention until it is too late, obviously the benefits are lost. I find it extremely helpful in encouraging practice to draw people's attention to potential situations where these techniques would be useful before the situations happen. The following activity helps direct your attention to situations where refocusing your emotional attention could improve a difficult situation or merely help you reach a higher potential.

In the space provided, brainstorm and list as many situations, both stressful situations and situations where higher functioning and clear coherent thinking would be highly desired, in which you could use these techniques. Remember, these techniques can be used right in the moment of stress, and no one ever even needs to know that you are making that shift. Even in a heated discussion, you can perform these steps and make an intentional internal shift without anyone being aware of what you are doing.

After listing as many situations that you can think of in the first column, list what for you are higher emotional states that you can intentionally cultivate in each situation. The cultivated higher emotional state may be specifically directed at that circumstance or situation, or it may not. Only you know what states will be conducive for you in specific circumstances. Also, it is important to remember that even if the cultivated internal state doesn't specifically match the situation, any improvement in your internal state will be beneficial. In other words, if you are in a situation where you are nervous, you may want to cultivate a state of calm or confidence. Or, you may feel more comfortable just making a shift to a peaceful state, or a state focused on gratitude or loving kindness. Only you know what is appropriate for you.

After listing situations and desired higher emotional states, in the third column list images that, for you, may help cultivate the desired emotional state. Remember, these are just tools to help you design a practice of refocusing your emotional attention to higher states. The shift is the most important aspect, and many specifics of the tools may change and evolve as you use them.

Situations	Desired Higher Emotional States	Images

Reflect and Process

Reflect and process about specific situations where these refocusing techniques may be helpful and the benefits you may receive from using them in these situations. Also, reflect on any specific ways you can remind yourself, right in the moment, to be able to make this shift. Write about images or things to help you remember and what images may work when. Reflect and process in a way that is beneficial to you. Explore your thoughts in some depth.

_____

_____

_____

_____

_____

_____

_____

_____

_____

_____

_____

_____

_____

_____

Where Is Your Attention?

These activities and tools to lead you through this process are only guides to help you cultivate your own practice of paying attention to and refocusing your emotional attention. The first and foremost challenge is paying attention to where your attention is in the first place. Teach yourself to routinely stop and notice where your emotional attention is. Cultivate the practice of being aware every moment of every day. Are you choosing to ruminate when it is not necessary? Are you choosing to catastrophize, when doing so will only create the physiological circumstances conducive to that catastrophe? Learn to stop and notice, refocus, and choose a higher emotional state.

Variations and Suggestions

Another beneficial way to use these techniques is to pick something about the situation that for you represents a higher emotional state, focus on that aspect, and allow yourself to feel it deeply. For instance, can you find something in a difficult situation for which you feel deeply grateful? If you examine this approach in light of what we know about the neuroscience and physiology of cultivating higher emotional states, it makes perfect sense. However, this technique will only work if you can really allow yourself to internally feel a sense of gratitude. Remember, it is the feeling state that creates the profound shifts in your physiology. Additionally, if you can perform the other steps of noticing and disengaging from your negative physical reaction, refocusing your physical attention by checking your eyes and shoulders, focusing your attention on your chest, and intentionally breathing, you will make the feeling shift to gratitude much more effectively.

You can adapt this concept to shift to any higher emotional state that works for you. One of my favorite ways to use this concept, the way that most resonates with me, is to connect with anyone involved in a difficult situation at the level of his or her soul or innermost being. The Quakers (and many other traditions, I'm sure) have a philosophy that you, me, and everyone carries the divine or utmost good at the deepest levels of themselves. It is present in everyone. The word *namasté* basically means that what is the divine essence in me salutes what is the divine essence in you. If I can recall this concept and acutely connect with this at a deep feeling level right in the moment, many difficulties are transformed. If I can disengage from the negative emotional reaction, refocus my physical attention, breathe deeply and sincerely, and connect at a feeling level with that divine essence, even when I'm angry or a specific behavior is not OK, I can proceed much more humanely, coherently, and clearly.

The Moment of Importance

By now, the benefits and possibilities of making an emotional shift right in the moment should be clear. We can make that shift in the moment of stress, we can make that shift at any moment we feel we could benefit from a higher potential, and we can make that shift using specifics from the circumstance. One of the most important aspects of making an intentional shift right in the moment is that it stops and reverses the stress process as it is occurring. Aside from the obvious fact of the enormous potential of influencing the outcome because your behavior is more clear, coherent, and functioning from a higher state, the physiological benefits are immediate.

Stressful responses are immediate. The biochemical reactions, including an influx of cortisol, the cardiovascular response in heart rate, blood pressure and heart rate variability, and shallow breathing, are instantaneous. Negative brain neural patterns and many more negative reactions flood the body as soon as we have the negative reactions. Most techniques, even positive techniques, to deal with stress usually require that we wait for an appropriate time.

For instance, when I ask students in my classes or seminars how they usually deal with stress, I get a wide variety of answers. Some cite negative things like smoking, drinking, eating, binge shopping, or other ways of self-medicating. Other cite positive practices like exercise, talking to a friend, yoga, meditation, and listening to music. The problem with all these practices, even the healthy ones, is that none can be done in the initial moment of the stress response.

The stress response in the body is immediate, but the physical effects may be long term and long lasting. Blood pressure may take a while to return to normal. Although adrenaline is a short-acting stress hormone, cortisol is not. Cortisol stays in the system for many hours, and once we have a higher level of circulating cortisol, it only takes a portion of that original level several hours later to return us to the level of the initial influx. In other words, cortisol is long lasting, repeated cortisol is even more damaging, and doing anything in the immediate moment to stop the influx or reduce its effects has immeasurable benefits.

If I wait to do something, even as beneficial as meditation, I am still carrying many of the physiological effects of the stress response until that time. Being able to refocus my emotional attention to a higher response and reactive pattern right in the moment of stress, I am profoundly changing the severity and the length of the negative experience. Once again, it is repeated experience and strength of experience that create and strengthen neural networks. If I allow myself to stay in a negative emotionally reactive place longer than is necessary, I am only training my body and brain to experience more of those states. If I routinely refocus my emotional attention to a higher state right in the moment of stress, I am profoundly changing my repeated experience.

We all have 24 hours in a day. How much of that time is your emotional attention in a negatively reactive place? How long is it focused on higher emotional states? How long do you carry around stressful events or reactive patterns stimulated by those events? Refocusing your emotional attention as you first notice a negative reactive pattern can save $23\frac{1}{2}$ hours of negative physiological and psychological experience.

Sustained Practice (Sustained HEART)

If experience creates and strengthens neural networks and biochemical response patterns, and repeated experience exaggerates this process, what we routinely and consistently expose ourselves to has a profound effect on who we are becoming at any point in time. Sustained practice of HEART provides the routine and consistent experience necessary for long-term change, or as Davidson says, the impetus necessary to raise our baseline level of happiness. Again, I don't claim that these techniques are any more beneficial than other sustained mental and emotional practices, but they are easy to use and offer an avenue to encourage those who might not otherwise adopt a sustained practice to do so.

This sustained practice is built on the concept that the longer and more routinely we expose ourselves to any physiological, psychological, or emotional state, the more likely our bodies are to adapt to that state and create it as our primary operating system. This concept works as exercise does. If we routinely and consistently create an internal experience, complete with the neural and biochemical shifts of a higher emotional state, our bodies adapt to that state by changes in structure and function.

When you routinely and consistently exercise, your body undergoes a complete overhaul of the way it functions. Muscles change, enzymes change, your cardiorespiratory system changes, and your use of blood sugar changes. If you have problems with high blood pressure, exercise may reduce it. Even your bones change. And these are only a few of the physiological changes taking place. In short, routine and consistent exercise transforms a body.

The same is true of sustained mental practice. But again, just as exercise must be experienced, so must mental practice. Sustained and routine practice of HEART will create fundamental changes in the operating system of the body and brain. Additionally, as Davidson found in his research on meditation practices, the more one practices, the more profound the changes. How then do we develop a sustained practice effective enough to produce those changes?

Information and advice for creating the external circumstances conducive to sustained and routine practice will be shared shortly, but let's look first at how the HEART can be modified from ease of use in the moment to ease of use for sustained and routine practice. Although the steps and physiological foundations of HEART are the same whether you use the techniques in the moment or as a sustained practice, some of the specifics are different.

To begin, it is important to have an environment conducive to sustaining an intentional higher emotional focus. Most of the time this means a quiet, comfortable place where you can sit uninterrupted and feel free to direct your emotional attention to a higher state. More will be shared on this shortly, but it is valuable to have this understanding as the steps are described in the context of sustained practice.

Additionally, it is essential to understand that by routine practice you are intentionally creating internal experience. This internal experience then produces the physiological and neural changes that have been the subject of most of this book. What is vital to understand about this intentional creation of inward experience is that the more routine the experience, the more profound are the physiological changes. Creating an environment supportive of sustained practice is imperative for the success of that practice.

In other words routine, consistency, and sustained practice are what produces change. What does all that mean in practical terms? Five to fifteen minutes a day will produce some positive changes. Twenty to thirty minutes once or twice a day will produce even greater benefits. When people are first beginning, unless they are very committed to creating a more serious practice, I suggest about fifteen minutes a day, as most people will perceive this amount of time as doable.

Another initial consideration is whether the use of music is conducive to your ability to focus your attention on higher emotional states. Some people prefer music, other prefer quiet. If you prefer music, the type of music you choose is very important. It must be slow and not too chaotic in its arrangement, as even some classical music can be. Some people also suggest that music with strong, dominant lyrics can be very distracting. The music must be perceived as background music and not occupy your conscious attention, which needs to be focused on intentionally creating a higher emotional state or holding an image that helps facilitate that state.

Musical accompaniments created specifically for this type of practice are available, but I suggest listening first to make sure they work for you. I have found that the use of music is quite individual and what works for one person may not necessarily work for another. There are musical scores intentionally created to match specific brain wave patterns that help facilitate a deeper experience. My favorite is by Jeffrey Thompson, a selection called *Brainwave Journey*. My students and participants in my seminars seem to respond positively to these musical scores, which are available in bigger music stores.

Once you have created a supportive environment and allotted an appropriate amount of time, follow the HEART steps with the following adaptations.

Begin by sitting in a comfortable position with your back straight. A straight back helps align your spine and gives room for your diaphragm to move. Your diaphragm is a muscle that cuts across your chest cavity, almost like a pancake. It is responsible, by its movement up and down, for creating pressure differences in your lungs that cause them to inflate and deflate. If your diaphragm doesn't have room to move, your lungs can't inflate sufficiently. Keep in mind how important the breathing process is to creating physiological change and refocusing your emotional attention.

In sustained practice, because we have more time and focused attention to contribute to the process, the steps should be deliberate with full emotional attention paid to each step.

Notice

The notice step in sustained practice is similar to HEART in the moment, but you might not be having an obvious negative physiological reaction as you do in the moment of the stress response. It is important to remember that sustained HEART is for the purposes of changing our baseline level of emotional functioning, and it is most like exercise in its conditioning aspect. Just because you may not be in the middle of a negative reactive response doesn't mean that practice is unimportant. Routine, sustained practice is vital in creating long-term physiological and neural change and in raising our baseline level of happiness.

The notice step in this practice requires you to take a brief inventory of the physical state of your body. Are your shoulders or any other areas of your body tight? Do you feel anxious? Pay attention to your physiological and psychological state, but don't get consumed in a reaction to that state. Scan your body. How does it feel? Are any areas harboring stress or tightness? How are you feeling generally from a psychological standpoint? Are there any feelings that stand out?

After you have physically and psychologically scanned your body, make a conscious effort to disengage from those feelings. If you have tightness or notice stress anywhere in your body, make a conscious effort to physically release that tightness. Sometimes it helps to visualize that part of your body and picture it relaxing or releasing the tension it is harboring. Another useful technique at this point is to repeat the word "release," either silently or aloud, as you breathe out and imagine yourself releasing any stress housed in your body.

Refocus

After you have scanned your body and disengaged from any negative physical or psychological reaction, make a conscious effort to release all the tension around your eyes. This step is similar to HEART in the moment, but you can apply much more conscious effort to releasing the tension and you can allow your eyes to close. Repeating the word "release" on the out breath, imagine the breath as leaving through your eyes to help facilitate this step. Remember that your eyes are powerfully connected to the emotional command center in your brain. Just by paying attention to and releasing the tension around your eyes, you're sending a powerful message to the command system in your brain to relax and calm your whole body.

After you have released the tension in your eyes, do the same with your shoulders. Release any tension, tightness, or stress in your shoulders, and repeat "release" on the out breath. Bring all your attention to an area of your chest that feels comfortable for you, whether you want to identify it as your heart, your solar plexus, the assemblage point, or just a comfortable area of your chest. Remember, bringing your conscious attention to an area in your chest physiologically helps turn off the area in the left temporal lobe of your brain that is responsible for constant chatter. Also, remember that this constant chatter perpetuates the stress response and negative emotional reactive patterns. Bringing your attention to a vital area in your heart or chest area helps you physiologically turn off the constant chatter of your brain and disengage from any negative response patterns.

Eyes, shoulders, chest. I think of this as stepping down to my heart. Once you have your conscious attention in a comfortable area of your chest, begin to breathe slowly, deeply, and comfortably. Recall all the positive physiological, biochemical, electrical, and neural responses to deep, slow breathing. They are numerous, and after routine practice, can be effective in establishing a new level of functioning for your emotional reactive patterns.

When you are at the breathing step of sustained HEART, your conscious attention is keenly focused at the area of your chest and on the process of breathing. It may be helpful to remind yourself to check your eyes and shoulders briefly to ensure they have remained relaxed, but, for the most part, your attention is acutely focused on your breathing. For some, it helps to repeat the word "release" on every out breath and vividly feel the sensation of releasing throughout your body, especially your eyes. Sometimes you hear this referred to as "breathing through your eyes." That's obviously impossible, but it does convey the intent of this step. Many traditions and practices recommend that you count each breath. Count each in-and-out cycle as one breath. Many people count from one to ten, and then go back to one, while others count down from ten to one and then go back to ten.

The idea of counting each breath is to help keep your attention keenly focused on your breathing and in the area of your chest. If your attention is keenly focused on your breathing, it won't be on anything else, like a negative emotional reactive state or the chatter of your brain. Another breathing tool I have seen some people use is to count 1-2-3 as you breathe in and 1-2-3 as you breathe out. Again the counting tools are just to engage your conscious mind enough to keep if from drifting off to another thought process and to keep it on the breathing process. The goal is not to really count how many times you have taken a breath, and if you find yourself on twenty-seven or thirty-five, just bring it back to one and begin again.

The main concept to remember when practicing these breathing tools and refocusing techniques is to do what works for you. Tailor your practice in a way that promotes the physiological changes discussed but in a way that feels comfortable and natural for you. The importance of breath in the refocusing process cannot be understated. Recall all the physiological implications and positive biochemical, electrical, and neural changes that intentional breathing promotes.

Choose _____

After several breathing cycles, with your attention keenly focused on your breathing, you will probably begin to feel a deep shift in both your physiological and psychological feeling states. Once you begin to feel this shift, make a conscious and intentional shift to a higher emotional state. Again, these states differ and evolve as your practice progresses, but you should use an image or feeling that intuitively feels comfortable for you at that time. The goal is to create a sincere feeling shift to a higher emotional state and induce all the positive physiological responses that go with that state. These physiological, biochemical, and neural responses are very real, very powerful, and they can create profound change if practiced regularly.

The main goal of sustained practice is to maintain the positive emotional shift long enough that you begin to make foundational shifts in your psychophysiology. Consequently, the important aspect here is that this state is genuinely sustained. It is not forced or faked, but is honestly experienced. If it is experienced enough, our bodies adapt with conditioned changes of internal experience.

In sustained practice our main purpose is to maintain this feeling state for a specified amount of time. If your mind begins to wander, gently bring it back to your practice. If holding an image helps you to create and maintain the feeling shift, it is a good tool to use. However, it is important to remember that the image is just a tool, and genuinely cultivating the feeling state is the important aspect of the practice. If you are holding an image, it is important to use an image that helps you make a shift to a higher emotional state. Occasionally, students or participants in my seminars try to use an image that they also associate with negative or sad emotions, and those emotions begin to surface during their practice. For instance, a participant wants to hold an image of a partner, but conflicted emotions from a negative experience in the relationship surface. Sometimes students who want to hold images of their grandparents become saddened because their grandparents have passed way and that sadness surfaces during their practice.

If you find yourself shifting from image to image, as participants new to practice often do, that is fine. The feeling shift is what matters, and you must use the image that works for you in that moment. It is also important to remember that the focus should be on sustaining a higher emotional feeling, so don't get caught up in a visual image that distracts you, as in an intricate daydream. As your practice becomes more developed and mature, you will find it is easier to cultivate feelings such as gratitude, loving kindness, compassion, and unconditional love, without necessarily holding an image. These states are the ones that have been shown to be the most beneficial though research.

If this still sounds foreign to you, recall the emotional charting exercise at the end of Chapter Five. Pick a higher emotional state that feels comfortable for you. If it helps to hold an image, pick an image that you can consciously hold in the cognitive part of your brain to induce a higher emotional reaction from the emotion control centers of the brain. The list you created at the end of Chapter Six may help you do this. Briefly review the HEART process. Find a comfortable quiet space in which to sit and, if you desire, play some soothing music.

Notice
- How you feel physically. Scan your body and make a conscious attempt to relax any area that is tight, stressed, or anxious.
- How you feel psychologically. Intentionally disengage from negative feelings.

Refocus
- Check your eyes and intentionally relax, then release on the out breath if it helps.
- Check your shoulders and intentionally relax them.
- Place all your attention at or around your heart or solar plexus.
- Breathe slowly and deeply, but most of all comfortably. Sustain this breathing, and use counting tools to keep your attention keenly focused. Vividly feel the sensation of release.

Choose _____
- When you begin to feel your body release, make an intentional shift to a higher emotional state and "feel" this state. Use an image if necessary.
- Sustain the relaxed breathing and focused emotional state for approximately fifteen minutes.
- If you find your mind wandering, gently bring your attention back and continue.
- Try to not get too caught up in the thought process and instead try to intentionally cultivate a nonconscious feeling state of a higher emotion.
- Sustain and breathe.

HEART Review

These Higher Emotion and Refocusing Techniques are intentionally and deceptively simple. A treasure of research supports the remarkable positive physiological and neural benefits of mental training focused on higher emotional states. In addition to the current research, there are many more hypotheses and theories that this type of training may produce even greater benefits, but because this area of research is so new, they have not yet been tested. However, the underlying science is sound, and it is my belief that it is only a matter of time before we realize even greater benefits.

These techniques were designed to be simple to encourage the routine experience of these practices necessary to create change. Our ultimate objective is to replace negative emotional reactive patterns with higher emotional reactions, and that can be done only through routine experience. Even the acronym HEART is designed as an easy reminder of the goal of the process. In times of stress or negative reactive states, go to HEART and your physiology, biochemistry, electrical and neural patterns, perception, and behaviors will change. The more authentically and sincerely you engage in the shift, the more powerful the changes will be. It is up to you.

In closing, I would like to review some important specific information to facilitate your ability to shift and create the routine internal experience necessary for change. Additionally, this chapter shares tools and particular practices that will enhance your success at creating those experiences. Most importantly, the answer lies in actually creating that internal experience. You need to move from "knowledge about" to "practice of," remembering that all experience creates or strengthens neural networks and biochemical reactions. If we are not actively creating those from intentional higher emotional states, we are probably unknowingly creating and strengthening those from negative emotionally reactive states.

I am deeply appreciative of all the work, knowledge, and research that has gone into the development of these techniques. Again, these techniques are not meant to claim superiority over any other practices. My purpose in developing these techniques is to take the phenomenal information we have learned regarding emotional and mental training and the plasticity of the brain and make it accessible, in an easily useable format, to those who would probably not otherwise practice.

HEART is designed to do in the moment of stress, in the moment you need to have a coherent reaction based on higher emotional states. It can also be used for sustained practice to promote long-term change in your baseline level of emotional functioning. I call these two uses *HEART in the moment* and *sustained HEART* for easy recall of their purposes. Although I have divided them into two distinct techniques, in reality their use should be thought of as a continuum. Anytime you can initiate HEART and intentionally focus your attention on a higher emotional state, you will benefit immensely. You will shift internally and become more at ease, you will think more clearly and become more productive, you will reach a higher potential for yourself and everyone around you.

HEART in the moment is designed to be done anytime, anywhere. The specific steps and physiological, neural, and biochemical implications have been shared in depth. Even though the steps were specifically separated, they are often done so quickly they almost seem simultaneous. Remember the specifics of each step, and practice as often as possible. Remember specific situations ahead of time where you are likely to benefit from their use. Routine practice will not only create fundamental changes in that moment, it will also help replace negative reactive patterns with positive ones.

Notice. Refocus. Choose _____.

The more you teach yourself to respond with an intentional higher emotional response, the more your body and psyche will automatically revert to this response as your typical experience. Experience creates changes in our physiological functioning. Once a new baseline level of emotional response is established, your body will regard this as the new norm and you will feel out of sorts if you respond in the old negative reactive patterns you once did.

Reminding yourself to make the shift is of fundamental importance. You are creating new experience by making the internal shift. If you don't remember to make the shift until it is too late, you have not only lost the opportunities to create change, you have solidified and strengthened negative reactive patterns. One phrase I think is valuable to commit to memory is "drop to your HEART." If, when you begin to feel a negative reactive pattern surfacing, you can remember this phrase, it will remind you to do the steps of HEART in the moment and begin to make an internal shift. Also, if by remembering that phrase you can recall all the physiological, neural, and biochemical implications of negative reactive patterns and the possibility of shifting those patterns with a different emotional focus, it should serve as motivation to practice the techniques.

Sustained HEART is designed to be used as routine and prolonged practice. When I presented the specific considerations of sustained practice, I encouraged you to identify a specific place conducive to practice. In fact, sustained practice of HEART is much more likely to be successful if you have identified a time and place in which to practice. Sustained practice is designed to create prolonged and consistent experience of higher emotional states. This prolonged and consistent experience will create more profound physiological changes because of the extended time in the higher experience. In other words, the more and longer you practice anything, the more likely change is to occur.

From extensive research in behavior change, and research in what it takes to motivate people to be consistent with any practice, we know if that it can become a habit a person is much more likely to perform and stick to that practice. Sustained HEART is like any other physiological practice, in that change won't occur unless it is routinely performed. So what does it take to make it a habit? We know that establishing a place conducive to practice is important. Only you can determine where this place is likely to be most effective, and some of us will have more trouble establishing an appropriate place then others.

Be creative and make it a priority. I have seen some so pressed for an appropriate place that they do it in their car. My practice has become so important to me I have a small room in my house dedicated to it. Before I had that luxury, I had converted a closet in my old house. I have seen some using any open church, even if they are not a member, and some people just using a random chair in their house. The place itself isn't as important as designating some place that encourages you to practice.

Time set in your schedule has also been shown to be an important component to successful behavior change or positive habit formation. If it is not set in your schedule, it is likely to get moved or replaced by other things on your to-do list. Make it a priority. Remember that positive changes happen from practice, but also that the negative reactive patterns we are accustomed to just become more ingrained if we do not make time to develop an alternative experience.

Social support and motivation are also very important aspects of behavior change. Social support and motivation are highly individual but necessary for success. Keep in mind these considerations, and develop a plan that is appropriate for you. I have been doing these practices long enough that my motivation has become that I now feel horrible when I don't practice. I like the feeling of calmness, clarity, and coherence I get from my practice, and this alone motivates me to continue.

Although specific arrangements for sustained practice are optimal, anytime, anyplace you can practice is beneficial. In a parked car, in a waiting room, under a tree, anytime you have a moment or anytime you want to think clearer, calm down, or refocus your emotional attention. Recall the mood congruency hypothesis. In these techniques you are using your conscious mind to stimulate the nonconscious mind to a higher emotional reaction. The mood congruency hypothesis states that what is stimulated in the emotional command center of our brain is congruent to where our current feeling attention is. Anytime you sincerely and genuinely practice refocusing your emotional attention to a higher state, you are more likely to create and sustain a more positive and higher functioning mood state.

Remember, there is a continuum of HEART, meaning that it doesn't always have to be the dichotomy of being purposely sustained or in the immediate moment. Many opportunities fall in between. You do not have to have your eyes closed; you do not have to be off by yourself. Anytime you can notice, refocus, and choose a higher emotional state, you will begin to shift your internal experience. After consistently and habitually bringing your attention to higher emotional states, you will begin to notice yourself routinely functioning from this calmer, more coherent state, feeling more empowered and reaching a higher potential. You will feel more equanimity in your own life, and this will be your new baseline level of functioning. You will actually strive to keep your attention on higher states, because when you do not, you will feel physiologically off-balance, and you won't like it.

When you are performing both HEART in the moment and sustained HEART, it is important to remember that each step is vital in the physiological, biochemical, electrical, and neural shifts that are taking place. At the end of the chapter will be a greatly simplified version of the steps. Commit it to memory. Each step, the order of the steps, and the process of disengaging from the negative emotional reactive state you are experiencing are all essential considerations in the refocusing process.

Images used to consciously induce nonconscious higher emotional reactions will vary, should vary, and are only tools to promote the desired result. The images usually vary from more simple (like my dog's face) to more complex (like the ecstasy I felt climbing Half Dome in Yosemite). Sometimes you may use images and sometimes you may not. Usually simple images work better in times of higher stress, or when you are more emotionally chaotic, and more complex images work when you are already feeling somewhat internally coherent. The most important thing to remember about the images is that the higher emotional state they induce is the vital component. You need to *feel* the reason why you hold that image dear.

The more you refocus your emotional attention to higher states, the more benefits you will gain by doing so. It is experience that creates change or strengthens existing patterns, and you are ultimately in charge of your internal experience. When you routinely experience higher emotional states, your body experiences internal coherence; that is, your body and brain work together more harmoniously and create physiological conditions more conducive of higher potential and higher functioning. Stopping and refocusing your emotional attention to a higher state at any time is beneficial.

With enough practice, our body establishes what Davidson described as a higher baseline level of happiness, or what I have referred to as a higher level of emotional functioning. This baseline becomes our new norm, or homeostasis, as we referred to it at the beginning of the book. When we reach a new level of homeostasis, our bodies and brains strive to keep this as our normal level of functioning, and we automatically make every effort to remain at this calm, coherent, and clear state.

When I first began teaching these concepts, one of my students adamantly wanted to know if I used these techniques myself, because he thought that would be the best indication of my belief in their validity. I could answer him with an unequivocal yes. I have used them consistently and reliably for many years. I do a sustained practice at least once a day for 25 minutes, and any time when needed, throughout the day. I used HEART, and still use it when I need to refocus my attention when I am writing and need to think more clearly. I use it in relationships with students, my partner, my children, and my friends. It has become an automatic reaction for me now—and for that I am truly grateful.

It would actually be easier to cite the times when I do not use HEART because now these concepts have become an ingrained part of who I am. I can say, without exaggeration, that there have been many times in my life in the last several years—involving external tragedies, major life events, or other key life challenges—when I honestly don't know how I would have made it through without my practice. My practice is a major foundation of my life and who I am.

Developing any physiologically based practice, whether it is exercise, meditation, or emotional refocusing techniques, relies on creating intentional experience to promote change. Experience is the key, and creating circumstances conducive to routine practice helps facilitate that experience. In other words, forethought and planning are required to create a follow through to experience. Change simply won't happen unless you engage in the activity.

How then do we use forethought and planning to follow through with emotional refocusing? Many psychologists identify specific phases of behavior change. The phases usually vary somewhat depending on what source you are referring to, but generally the first three steps are pre-contemplation, contemplation, and action. Pre-contemplation is basically when you are oblivious to a need or possibility of change. Contemplation begins when you identify a need or desire for change and begin to make plans for that change. Action is when you engage fully in the activity to promote change.

It is my experience that most people desiring change get stuck in the contemplation phase. They are constantly making plans for change, but never really fully engage in the action phase, therefore never fully reaping the benefits. More will be said in the next chapter about reasons why this might be true, but for now let's entertain the need for specific plans. When specific plans are made for actions, those actions are more likely to succeed and become experience. More simply, if we know who, what, where, when, and how, as specifically as possible, we are more likely to actually engage in the proposed action.

One important step for refocusing your emotional attention in the moment was represented in Activity/Reflection #7. Being aware ahead of time of any situation that you are likely to benefit from cultivating a higher emotional state will help you follow through with that intention when the situation arises. In the following reflection you will further examine potential situations that may benefit from higher emotional attention. It is important to remember that refocused emotional attention is not only appropriate for times when you feel the emotional unease associated with stress, anxiety, conflict, or fear. Refocusing your attention to a higher emotional state, because of the powerful biological implications, will also help you *routinely* function from a higher emotional state and reach higher potential and greater productivity.

Additionally, it is extremely important to grasp the fact that experience creates and strengthens neural networks and biochemical reactive patterns, even if that experience is negative. If we are not actively working to create positive intentional shifts in our reactive patterns, we are probably falling victim to ingrained negative reactive patterns and strengthening those patterns. We need to internalize that we can use these concepts as a foundation for a way of living that helps us feel clear, inspired, and internally coherent, and the more we incorporate these concepts into our lives, the more change we are likely to see and feel. Like exercise, the more focused attention, time, and effort we spend engaging in creating an alternative experience, the more we will undergo transformation.

"Cheat Sheet" for HEART

HEART in the Moment

Notice— Catch your physical and psychological reactions to any negative event the moment they happen.

Intentionally disengage from those reactions.

Refocus— Check and release:

Your eyes

Your shoulders

Bring your attention to a comfortable spot in your chest.

Engage in slow, deep, intentional breathing.

Choose— Let yourself shift to, and feel, a higher emotional state. If it helps, use an image to facilitate this shift, or pick something about the situation for which you can feel grateful. Keeping your eyes and shoulders relaxed, and your attention at your chest and your breathing, maintain the higher emotional state as long as is appropriate.

Sustained HEART

Find a quiet place where you can engage in a genuine and sustained shift to a higher emotional state. Sit straight enough to allow your diaphragm room to move and your lungs room to fully inflate.

Notice— How you feel physically and psychologically. Intentionally disengage from these feelings if they are negative.

Refocus— Check your eyes and shoulders, and intentionally release any tension.

Place your attention at a comfortable spot in your chest.

Breathe slowly and deeply, but most of all comfortably. Maintain, count your breaths, and feel the sensation of release throughout your body.

Choose— When you begin to feel your body release, make an intentional shift to a higher emotional state and "feel" this state. Use an image, if necessary. Sustain for approximately 15–20 minutes. If you find your mind wandering, gently bring your attention back and continue.

HEART in Action
ACTIVITY AND REFLECTION #8

This chapter focuses on intentionally cultivating higher internal experiences. The techniques presented here are designed to help you routinely and consistently do that. It is my experience that the more I can encourage people in forethought of what that might "look" like for them, the more successful they will be. Following are several questions for reflection to encourage deeper engagement of the concepts presented. Again, this practice needs to be your own, and the more you can internalize the personal aspects of it, the more effective your practice will be.

Brainstorm, reflect, and write on the following two pages. Think about how you can most effectively engage these concepts in your own life. Following are questions to ponder. They are designed to stimulate thought on your part about what would be the most effective ways to use and put into practice these concepts in your own life.

Review what for you feels like a higher emotional state. What resonates most with you? What does the word *gratitude* feel like? Or *compassion*? Or *understanding*? Or any other higher state that is more appropriate for you? Review the images you have described that may elicit those feelings for you. Do these images need to be modified in any way?

How can you best train yourself to be conscious of where your attention is? How can you train yourself to find something to be grateful for in a challenging situation? Examine some of these situations in your life. What can you be grateful for in those situations? We all have 24 hours in a day. How much of that time is your emotional attention in a negatively reactive place? How long is it focused on higher emotional states? How long do you carry around stressful events or reactive patterns stimulated by those events?

How can you create an environment conducive to sustained practice? Where will you practice? Practice is much more successful if it is built into your schedule. How, specifically, will you build it into your schedule? Be specific about dates, places, and times. How else can you create a supportive environment to encourage practice?

These questions are meant to direct your thinking, not to be answered verbatim. Reflect, ponder, contemplate, and consider. How can you effectively cultivate higher internal experience, routinely and consistently, specifically and generally, in your own life?

_____

_____

_____

_____

Journal of Practice

I have found that through extensive experience teaching about and presenting these concepts, the value of a record sheet of practice cannot be understated. A record sheet of practice is an incredibly valuable tool in making the transition from contemplation to action. The record sheet of practice reminds you to put the techniques into your daily awareness and actually engage in using them. Again, practice is what makes the difference between "knowledge of" and "sincere engagement in," the latter of which is the prerequisite for shifting internal experience.

Another reward of keeping a record of practice is the insights that can be gained from doing so. Recording routine practice not only gives you valuable insight of what you might have learned through each cultivated experience, the cumulative knowledge is also very useful. You begin to see patterns emerge, you begin to see growth, and it may be a useful tool in evolving your personal practice.

Having my students and participants keep records of practice has helped them see growth throughout the process, and solidified their commitment to use the techniques because they are able to see consistent results; sometimes if you don't record the experience right away, you forget about it. On the following page is a log intended for you to record each experience. How you record is a matter of personal preference. Sometimes you may want to write more about any insights you had, how a circumstance was influenced by using these techniques, or what worked for you and what didn't. Record all experiences, including HEART in the moment and sustained HEART. Also, if you do any other practice that involves shifting internal experience, it would be valuable to record those experiences as well.

Remember these techniques were developed for ease of use and as an easy reminder of the power of intentionally cultivating higher emotional states. Any practice that encourages a shift to higher emotions and facilitates that process is appropriate to be included on this list. It may be conscious connection, it may be focused gratitude, or it may be any other sustained practice in which you routinely engage. The point is that higher internal experience is the goal, and recording that experience can enhance its further development.

Record Log

Date and record any time you have specifically engaged in HEART, either sustained or in the moment, and reactions and reflections of that experience. Also, if it is appropriate, record any other experiences in which you have engaged in an intentional shift to a higher emotional state. Examples include sustained practice in yoga, meditation, spiritual music or dancing, or intentional conversation and connections. Enter a date, record the event, and write any reflections you may have regarding the event.

_____

_____

_____

_____

_____

_____

_____

_____

_____

_____

_____

_____

REFERENCE

1. Begley, S., *Train Your Mind, Change Your Brain: How a New Science Reveals Our Extraordinary Potential to Transform Our Lives* (New York: Ballantine Books, 2007).

CHAPTER nine

Authentic Willingness

Are You Willing?

What prevents most people from substantial change? I believe they do not have a true willingness to live differently. In our journey to this point, we have explored stress and anxiety and concluded that what best characterizes these states is a feeling of emotional unease. We have looked at the process of emotion. Through our examination of the process of emotional reactive patterns, we have seen the absolute damage we do to ourselves when we allow ourselves to keep our attention in negative states, to create catastrophes in our thoughts, and to ruminate or constantly function from lower emotional states, including fear, guilt, hatred, and jealousy.

We have seen, through an in-depth physiological examination, the tremendous possibilities for our bodies, brains, and psyches and the resultant improvements in perceptions, behaviors, and relationships by intentionally cultivating higher emotional states. We have explored one specific group of techniques based on physiological, biochemical, and electrical foundations and designed to facilitate and encourage cultivating those states. We have determined, again through the process of physiology, that it is our repeated internal experience that determines our reactive patterns, creates and strengthens our neural networks, and influences our biochemical and electrical reactions. We have determined that the feeling state of our attention is primarily responsible for our internal experience, and the specific techniques presented in this book are aimed at shifting that "feeling attention" to higher emotional states. We have even worked through the process of what constitutes effective behavior change, examined our own personal experiences in light of that change, and developed specific plans of how to implement these techniques in our lives.

All that remains is to *want* change, to want to reduce the stress, chaos, and anxiety in your life and live from a more internally coherent, peaceful, and happy place. Many people profess to do so, but most are not willing to allow themselves to live differently. The stress, chaos, and anxiety have become such familiar states that, I believe, people are really not willing to replace them with higher functioning states, states with a higher baseline of happiness and full of higher potential. These questions are not just about reducing the stress and anxiety in our lives—indeed, some of you reading this may profess that you're not troubled by stress or anxiety—but about living the lives we were meant to live.

Higher functioning states. Higher potential. A higher baseline level of happiness and higher emotional states. After reading all these terms, it should be obvious that the connecting thread throughout them is the word *higher*. We have previously referred to an article by Astin and Keen on equanimity, or the ability to authentically see the silver lining. The article cites substantial research on the benefits of feeling good, feeling at peace, and feeling a "strong connection," all states I would associate with higher emotional states. These are feeling statements, not thinking statements, and the internal experience of these statements likely activates the limbic portion of the brain.

But does it stop there? Astin and Keen assert, and I agree, that these feeling states are associated with what we usually associate with higher states of consciousness.[1] Calm, centeredness, self-transcendence, compassion, kindness—intentionally cultivating these feeling states leads to higher potential, a higher baseline level of happiness, higher functioning states, and ultimately higher consciousness. Do these higher states of consciousness originate in our limbic system or from a higher source? I personally believe that they come from somewhere other than ourselves, that our limbic system is a reflection of the internal experience of these states rather than the original source. However, whether you agree with me or not, intentionally cultivating these states can profoundly change your brain, your body, and the way you function in the world. Beyond that, they may even lead you to higher states of consciousness.

Still the question of willingness looms large. As we continue our journey, we return to the question of willingness. It is my belief that although most people profess to want change, growth, transformation, or even higher states of consciousness, they are not really willing to accept these things in their lives. Transformative information and resources abound, and yet, I believe that at a fundamental level, people are not ready or willing or they lack the courage to truly embrace positive change. This positive change must come from within. It is the internal experience that gives meaning to and creates the external experience.

Any book or program aimed at positive transformation must address the question of true willingness. If we do not address this question, we remain in the contemplation stage instead of the action stage of behavior change. Contemplation of change will not propel us forward or inward. Only action will. As difficult as this question of willingness is, it must be addressed. Unfortunately, many people wait for tragedy or crisis to strike before they are willing to change.

The question of willingness applies at many different levels. It applies to major change. It applies to change to remove ourselves from status quo and grow out of the stress and anxieties that consume us. It applies when we are comfortable where we are but desire to reach a higher potential.

This chapter addresses the questions of willingness and allowance. Are we really ready to allow ourselves to drop our habitual ways of thinking and reacting and thus create a different internal experience? Are we willing to function from a different internal paradigm? Are we willing to take the internal and external steps necessary to create change? Are we willing to drop the paradigm that external success is the only measure of success and that cultivating positive internal experience will actually lead us to a higher potential than external experience alone?

Internal vs. External Experience

The world is full of those who have created external experience or success that our culture deems noteworthy and are still not allowing themselves to be happy. Unfortunately, at the time I write this, Americans tune in daily to media reports of young famous females whose lives are falling apart because they are internal messes. They are exhibiting out-of-control behavior, including drunk driving, overt drug use and abuse, public displays of inappropriate and damaging behavior, and even suicide. Over and over again, we have seen what we deem as culturally thriving successes in the form of movie stars, successful musicians, and other public figures self-destruct internally. In fact, our cultural history is flooded with icons who died young because they were elevated to the status of external success without developing the internal integrity to live up to those expectations.

I do not use the word *integrity* in a judgmental or harsh way. My friend John at the coffee shop, an extremely wise man whom I greatly admire, says integrity comes from internal integration. Acting out of integrity, then, comes from acting and behaving from an internally coherent state. Again, we return to the fundamental importance of internal experience.

Although these cultural icons are the most prominent in our minds, this scenario plays itself out over and over again throughout our society. We all know people who strive and strive for, and may even be successful at obtaining, what our culture deems as either monetary or career-related success. It is almost as if it is our belief that with enough external notoriety, a positive internal experience will naturally follow. The prevalent belief seems to be "if society says I'm OK, then I must be OK." Of course this is a never-ending push because the internal acceptance that is expected to follow doesn't appear, or it merely isn't regarded, and even great success leaves people feeling empty.

My point is not that external success and acceptance is not important. However, remember that it is our limbic system that creates internal experience and gives meaning to circumstance. If our internal experience isn't integrated with our external success, that success is void of meaning. The internal must come first. The internal gives meaning to and creates the external. If your goal is to be externally successful, for that success to be meaningful or lasting, it must first come from within. Higher internal experience creates higher potential, empowerment, and intention, and if external success is your goal, it will naturally flow from an internally integrated state. Returning to a metaphor we used in Chapter One, when you bring your attention to the right wall (meaning higher internal experience), the ladder appears.

Internal willingness is the true question. We have the knowledge. The first part of this book, along with a wealth of other books and research, gives us that knowledge. We have the practical steps of creating higher internal experience. Many practices abound, including the specific techniques presented in this book, that lead us through the process of elevating our internal experience to achieve real and measurable changes in our physiology. We even have created, through the activities in the last chapter, a step-by-step plan to help us implement this process. So, why don't we? What's the payoff in staying stuck? Are we truly willing to live differently?

Are You Ready to Allow?

So far, the discussion of willingness and allowance has focused on those terms as vague, general, and abstract constructs. What do those words really mean in practical, applicable terms? What does *willingness* really mean? What does *allowance* mean? What is the difference between those two terms? Why do we argue that we want change, and yet the real possibility of it feels physically uncomfortable? What are the payoffs in staying stuck, and how do we effectively apply these concepts to get unstuck? The answers to these questions—and how we can concretely apply the concepts of willingness and allowance in our own lives—are the focus of this chapter.

When I look up the word *willing* in various dictionaries, the main description or definition that keeps reappearing is the word *ready*. When I do the same for the word *willingness,* the main definition that comes up is "ready to do something." When I look up the word *allow,* I get the definition "give permission for something to happen," and the most fitting definition for *allowance* is "allowing something to happen."

What do those terms mean when we apply them to cultivating a higher internal experience? If we are talking about internal experience, then we need to examine the concept of being willing or ready from a deeply authentic or innermost place of awareness. In other words, are we really ready, from the deepest parts of who we are, to be or behave differently? Are we really ready to allow, or give permission, for the concepts presented throughout this book to play a part in our lives?

At this point I think most readers would say yes. However, when we dig even deeper and get more specific, that affirmative answer may change. For instance, the next time you have a negative reactive pattern and you react out of fear, jealousy, or hatred, consider whether you are really willing to react differently by functioning from a higher emotional state. Will you give yourself permission to truly let go of your negatively ingrained reactive patterns and replace them with cultivated states of higher consciousness? Are you really ready and willing to do the sustained practice that it takes, either the practice proposed in this book or another, to transform your reactive states to those based on higher awareness and higher potential?

An idea from Marianne Williamson is quite fitting at this point:

Our greatest fear is not that we are inadequate, but that we are powerful beyond measure. It is our light, not our darkness that frightens us. We ask ourselves who am I to be brilliant, gorgeous, handsome, talented and fabulous? Actually, who are you not to be? . . . Your playing small does not serve the world . . .

We seem to think we are ready and willing, in an external sense, to receive and strive for our highest potential. However, what we really need to examine is if we are willing, from an internal sense, to create the conditions necessary for those things to become manifest. We think we want those things, but are we really ready to stop sabotaging our efforts and create the internal circumstances necessary to receive? Are we really ready to stop perpetuating status quo?

Some will answer no. The status quo is perfectly fine for them because they believe it is an adequately functioning state. This question is not directed at them. This question is directed at those who profess to want change, those who profess to want to reduce the stress, chaos, and anxiety in their lives and live lives of higher potential. This question is for those who desperately want to live calmer, more internally coherent lives. What we need to examine in our exploration of willingness is what is keeping us stuck and how we can take concrete steps to get unstuck.

What's Keeping You Stuck? Examining the Payoff

Two main concepts stand out for me when I examine the question of what keeps us stuck. The first is the consideration of the payoff in staying stuck. If there are areas of your life you feel you would like change, you must be open to a sincere assessment of your willingness and true internal readiness. That includes an exploration of the "advantages" of staying stuck. In all situations there are positives and negatives, and honestly looking at the advantages of staying at status quo may be the key to understanding. You may examine a specific situation in your life and, after identifying and comparing the advantages and disadvantages of change, determine that change for you right now is not worth the effort. Or, you may decide that you prefer change—and this honest examination of the payoffs of staying stuck is what you needed to do to be able to move on.

The payoffs can be tangible or more psychological. Many times the psychological payoff, unfortunately, is that it feeds into your perceptions of being a victim. In other words, you're not willing to let go of a specific thought or feeling because it is a feeling you feel entitled to because in your mind someone has wronged you. Tangible or intangible, if you are not aware of the payoffs, you may not be able to move beyond them. But ultimately, whether or not you decide it is time for change, you need to honor yourself in the process.

Some examples may make these points more clear. One of my students professes to want major change in his life. He is an older student who lives with a parent and doesn't have a job. He doesn't like himself because he feels he doesn't have the internal resources to move on. The payoff for him is that the status quo is a comfortable existence, he doesn't have to work through the discomfort of growth, and it plays into his perception of himself as being incapable of moving on.

A participant in one of my seminars has had to deal with some tough issues in her life, and these have left her with some psychological reactive points. She makes statements like "That's just what my husband used to do," rationalizing or insinuating that "therefore I am entitled to this reaction." The payoff for her is she stays stuck in her perception of the circumstances that have influenced her. In other words, her perceptions reinforce the negative image of how bad things always happen to her and how people always wrong her. Recognizing that this is in some way a payoff, but a negative payoff, is the first step in being able to move on from those perceptions.

There are certain circumstances in my own life where I had thought I wanted change in a specific area, but after examining the situation in its totality, including the payoffs in staying stuck, I decided that I needed to wait until I was truly willing. Conversely, examining the payoffs and genuinely deciding they are worth giving up serves as motivation for change. Professing to want change, without a true examination of willingness, only increases our stress and blocks us off from our internal selves. Only when an examination of willingness leads us to an affirmative and receptive yes are we ready to authentically allow change to happen.

These are just a few brief examples. All people in many, many, different situations in their lives have multiple areas to question authentic willingness. You might find yourself rationalizing "this is the way I've always been," "this is because of my childhood," or "this is what my former partner (or parent or sibling or child) used to do." If you are using these rationales as a reason to stay stuck, you might question your willingness for change. Obviously, some people have deep psychological wounds, and this discussion is not intended to demean them. But if you truly desire to move beyond those wounds, you need to be willing to let them go. You need to examine if you are truly willing to allow a different perception of yourself, and you need to routinely replace your reactive patterns with those of higher emotional states—to choose to react with love instead of fear, to choose to react with compassion instead of fear or guilt, to choose to honor the sacred in all you encounter.

The Physiological Discomfort of Change

The second reason we choose to remain stuck is physiological discomfort of change. As was shared throughout much of this book, we have specific biochemical reactions to negative emotions. The biochemicals flood our bodies and brains, and it is as if our cells actually become addicted to that biochemical state. If fear and anger keep us in a specific biochemical state, and our cells crave that biochemical state because it is familiar, we want to keep experiencing fear and anger because it feels comfortable. Conversely, it actually feels physiologically uncomfortable to be willing to let those states go and replace them with positive states, even though they are much more coherent and healthy states. It all comes back to routine experience. If we routinely experience negative reactive states, then those states are what we become addicted to and we crave to stay in those states. However, if we routinely experience higher emotional states, which we can intentionally cultivate, then those states are what we become addicted to and we crave to stay in those states.

Willingness in this sense may be the understanding and awareness that there is a new biochemical reactive pattern to establish, and it takes willingness to adopt reactive patterns that establish those states. This concept is of fundamental importance in creating internal higher experience. Are you really willing, in the middle of a negative reactive pattern, to replace the lower emotional states with higher ones? Are you willing to let go of the perception that you have the right to react in a specific manner because that's "just the way you feel"? Are you really willing to let go of reactive patterns that are built on past negative experience and not assign that reactive pattern to the current circumstance? Are you willing to let go of your justified righteousness and replace that reaction with a calm, coherent, clear, and empowering response?

Reactive patterns create biochemical responses, and biochemical responses create reactive patterns. Are you willing, from a fundamental level, to notice and disengage from your reactive patterns as they happen, refocus your attention, and choose a reaction based on a higher emotional state? Unless you are truly willing to allow yourself to respond differently, the negative reactive patterns encoded in your brain will never transform. Unless you are genuinely willing to allow yourself a different reaction, your internal experience will remain the same. Are you willing to give your brain and body an alternative positive experience from which to grow?

One of the most transformative and important experiences I have had dealing with these concepts is in my relationship with my children. We were going through an especially rough period—not uncommon with two teenage boys—and I found myself much more frustrated and angry than usual. Of course this frustration and anger only made the situation a whole lot worse, but I felt completely justified by those responses as they were making some very poor choices. Just at the point I felt completely overwhelmed, I decided to try an experiment.

Every day for the first ten minutes when I woke up, and most often during my daily sustained practice, I would completely focus on and literally bathe myself in the gratitude I feel for my children. Admittedly, at first this was hard to do because of their current behavior, but I was persistent in my practice. Even though that practice was seemingly unrelated because it was at a different time of the day than when we were having difficulties, our relationship at that point began to transform. I found myself reacting, more often than not, from a caring stance, and my positive reactive behavior began to stimulate a change in their behavior.

They could feel the love, gratitude, and care I felt for them, and they responded positively. Because a good deal of my attention was on care, I could set down caring and safe guidelines instead of angry reactive ones, and we all transformed in our relationship. The power in that change was obvious and truly the only initial behavior change was in my sustained focus of gratitude, but I could feel the difference. My reactive patterns were profoundly changed, and we more often began to operate from love and care as the foundation of the relationship than from the opposite.

The Importance of Physiology

This book is founded on the concept that by intentionally cultivating physiological shifts in our brains and bodies, we can develop higher states of consciousness and, in doing so, change the circumstances by which we live. Another significant area of this concept is in dealing with challenging and specific issues or situations. In other words, imagine a specific issue or situation that is especially challenging for you. Examine your willingness to truly work through the situation from a higher state of consciousness. If you are truly willing, and you can feel what it would feel like to be done with or at a more positive point in the situation, you have already begun to make the physiological shifts conducive to solving that issue.

You see this phenomenon play out in sports training. One of my heroes, to whom I am honored to be very close personally, is a man named John Scolinos. "Coach" is a college baseball coach and was voted national collegiate baseball coach of the century. His teams won four national championships in ten years. Coach would spend almost as much time with his athletes in mental training for the game as he would in physical training. Every player was required to read and carry copy of *Psycho-Cybernetics* by Maxwell Maltz and constantly and consistently practice visualization. Visualization and intentionally cultivating higher emotional states are different practices, but they do overlap.

One of the areas that I believe has evolved about the process of visualization and the difference between it and intentionally creating feeling states is the discoveries in neuroscience that the feeling aspect is all important. In *Psycho-Cybernetics,* which is at this point a quite dated book, Maltz recommends that during the process of visualization, you vividly imagine all the details and feelings associated with the visualized experience. I believe that by his recommendation of attention to detail, he actually encouraged the experience of the feeling state. I also believe that the current discoveries in neuroscience prove what we have known about effective visualization.

Coach Scolinos coached the first Olympic baseball team in 1984. He tells a story of a discussion he had with gymnast Mary Lou Retton after her perfect 10. He asked her what she attributed her success to, and she said practicing visualization. For her to win the gold medal that day, she could have performed nothing less than a perfect 10. Most people thought that was impossible, yet she performed perfectly, won the gold, and attributed the success to her mental training. For successful athletes, willingness doesn't seem to be a problem. What about circumstances in daily life where we have a specific perception of our abilities that limits our growth?

One of my sons has had major growth points in his life that demonstrate this concept. Learning to ride a bicycle and learning to snowboard were quite traumatic events initially, complete with tantrums and emotional upheavals. In both of these circumstances I knew he was capable of the activity, but he was not ready to perceive himself as someone who could do those things. In both of those cases, the moment he was willing to perceive himself differently (one was prompted by a "magic push" from my father) was the moment he succeeded. In both instances he performed as if he had been doing the activity for years. The moment he could see himself differently was the moment he began to create the physiological changes necessary for success. Ask yourself what it would really "feel" like to already be in the condition or conditions you want to create, or free of the unease you want to shed. Just being willing to feel those states begins to create the physiological conditions necessary for change.

What do these stories have to do with willingness? The moment you are truly willing and able to release the negative reactive patterns associated with a situation and replace those negative reactive patterns with a positive feeling shift, you create the physiological conditions conducive to solving that situation. It's as if your brain believes you have already created those external conditions and begins to act accordingly.

The significance of this point cannot be understated. Are you willing to really see yourself in a position of already achieving the change you desire? This concept is vastly different from "wanting" something. When you want something but can't allow yourself to make the physiological shift to feeling what it would genuinely feel like to receive it or achieve it, you perpetuate the physiological condition of lack.

Again we begin with the higher internal experience that creates our physiological shift. Many people talk about this concept as intention or attraction. This book is full of the physiological rationale of why intention and attraction work. We begin at the level of our physiology and create the conditions necessary to make that intention a reality. The moment you are truly willing to make this authentic internal shift is the moment the shift begins to take place.

How, concretely, do we develop genuine willingness and allowance to cultivate higher emotional states? To address that question we will consider general concepts and practical applications and end with specific questions to examine our own level of willingness and allowance. Remember, our working definitions are of willingness as being authentically ready for and allowance as permitting inner change.

Fear and Reluctance

Taking a general look at willingness and allowance requires us to return to the concept of the ineffable. If we are defining willingness as being ready for growth or change and allowance as permitting that change to take place, we are looking at concepts that are hard to put into words. These concepts apply to small and large change and to differing degrees of transformation. Some choose to grow rapidly in spurts, and others choose to grow slowly over long periods of time. There is no one correct way, except what is appropriate for you.

One concept that borders on the ineffable regarding willingness to change is the fear that may accompany that growth. Most of us, when we are stuck, don't want to admit that there may be fear associated with that change, so change is kept at an external level of experience. However, if we look at the internal experience as what creates our reality, we must also take a deep look at the fear or reluctance, which may be subconscious, of change. If we do not at least entertain this reluctance, we easily sabotage our own efforts at change.

Part of willingness involves the discomfort of growth. Even if it is positive growth, there may be some aspect of fear of the unknown or fear of growing out of the familiar. Understand that this is part of the process. What is it about change that scares us? Is it the fear of the unknown? Is it that, although we may not like the current circumstance that we are trying to change, we are accustomed to it?

We see reluctance to accept change in our culture. We see reluctance to change physiologically. We need to take an honest look at our own reluctance or fear at a very deep level before we are truly ready to embrace the desired change. Otherwise, we will think we want it but probably fall back into our old patterns and way of doing things. Unfortunately, most efforts at many types of personal change have proven unsuccessful statistically in the long run. I believe this is because the internal experience of change hasn't mirrored the external.

Our culture seems to limit change. Many times it is hard for those around us to feel comfortable with personal growth, because this growth somehow may change the dynamics of the usual ways of functioning within the "system." Also, our culture in many ways denounces personal change, especially for those a little older, as evidenced by phrases like "she's going through her second childhood," or "mid-life crisis." Just the semantics of these terms hold a severely judgmental tone.

During an internally transformative period of his life, my brother fielded many pointed questions about whether he might be going through a mid-life crisis. He mused, "If this is a mid-life crisis, bring it on!!" I reflected on that concept quite a bit and on the influence of semantics. Why don't we call it a mid-life *transformation*? This would have been especially appropriate in my brother's case because his transformation was full of extremely positive internal change. We seem to have this culturally mandated judgment that personal change is somehow a sign of weakness or escape. I sincerely believe transformative experience should be embraced, and if these experiences were not looked down upon by our culture, they would more likely be laced with positive internal growth rather than external "grabbing." I also believe, because of the reluctance of our culture to embrace transformation, that's where people get off track with something like a mid-life crisis. If our culture would embrace and encourage change, people would work to fill the void with nurturing and positive internal transformation rather than an external "toy."

The question of fear of or reluctance to change is difficult. Most will deny any fear and say they just want change. As hard as these questions may be, they must be at least entertained to experience deep and lasting change. If you just want change, why haven't you achieved it yet? There may not be answers in words, just a recognition that on some level fear or reluctance exists. The answers don't have to be in words; simple recognition can help us move on. If we are willing and able to identify the barriers in words, these realizations can help us take concrete action to remove those barriers and proceed.

The fear may be merely the ineffable fear of the unknown or unfamiliar. Recognition of that feeling helps us move on, or not, and be OK in that space. I love the metaphor of a car driving through the dark. When a car travels in the dark, only the car's headlights light the road. Those headlights shine only about 200 feet in front of where the car is traveling, but those 200 feet are always enough, as long as the car is traveling at a safe speed for the conditions. When I feel the fear of growth and I know I need to experience some sort of transformation, I can ground myself in that metaphor. Then, I am a little more at ease with the fear of the unknown. I know that I will see what I need to see as it is appropriate, and if I can stay centered in my own internal experience, that transformation will come.

One of the absolute best practices to keep grounded in the internal experience of change and not be consumed with some nonspecific fear or sabotaging your own efforts is to keep a personal journal throughout the process. The journal will help keep you grounded, centered, and focused on what change feels comfortable for you.

When I was going through a transformative period in my life, I remember talking to a friend about very strong, but nonspecific, fears about the process and about being afraid to get caught up in old patterns that would limit me. He bluntly asked me if I could just not change. I thought for a moment and genuinely said, "No." I was aware I wanted and needed this growth, and I would never be happy if I didn't follow the path.

In the conclusion to this chapter, I address many questions. These questions are as important as any text in this chapter. I choose to present these concepts in the form of questions as to not dilute the difficult and important process of deep willingness with too many words. Do not skim over these questions. Read each, internalize the concept, and address their importance in your own life. A large part of authentic willingness borders on the ineffable. We can understand what genuine willingness feels like but it is hard to put into words. Read these questions from that state.

Read each question and pause. Tune into that part of your chest that seems to hold the answers for you. Remember that not all these questions are meant to be answered affirmatively. Change must come in a way and at a rate that feels comfortable for you. Again, some people seem to change slowly over long periods of time, and other change rapidly in bursts of growth. Honor what feels right for you and honor when an answer is no. Most of all, keep in mind the scientific and physiological principles behind authentic willingness, and know that when you are truly willing, change will take place.

General Questions of Willingness

1. Are you really willing and ready for internal change or transformation in small or large ways? (No is OK.)

2. Much of this book has been on the process of negative reactive patterns and identifying personal trigger points. Are you truly willing to examine your own trigger points, "own them," and work to let them go?

3. We all have emotional baggage. My friend likes to say, "If we don't unpack our emotional baggage here, we'll just have to carry it awhile longer." Are you willing to admit to your emotional baggage? Are you willing to "unpack" it and let it go?

4. Are you truthfully willing to examine your perceptions of events and whether those perceptions are based on higher emotions or negative based reactive patterns? Are you willing to allow yourself a different subjective interpretation of routine events that will allow you to experience a higher level of happiness, acutely remembering the physiological adaptations that are happening with either interpretation?

5. Are you willing to let go of thoughts like "that's just the way I feel" or "that's just my perception," when in truth you are using those statements to validate or wallow in a negative reactive pattern?

6. Are you willing to recognize and work through the discomfort of change and allow yourself a new paradigm as a way of being?

7. Are you willing to stay grounded throughout this process by keeping a journal or collection of personal reflective writing?

Questions of Practice

Much of the preceding chapters were devoted to the physiological foundations and specific techniques to refocus your emotional attention to higher states. The physiological foundations are sound. What is the necessary and quite often missing ingredient is true and authentic practice. These techniques are the most potentially transformative information in this book, as they are what change us at the physiological level. However, they simply will not work if they are not engaged. The following questions address the question of willingness to do what it takes to promote deep change at the physiological level, which, in turn, changes our existence.

1. Are you willing to do what it takes to remind yourself you have a different way to respond when you feel a negative reactive pattern surfacing based on anger, guilt, frustration, or anxiety?

2. Are you truly willing in the moment of a negative reactive pattern to disengage yourself from that pattern and choose a reaction based on higher emotional states?

3. Are you genuinely willing to do a routine sustained practice of mental training or cultivating higher emotional states or higher states of consciousness? Are you willing to set up a program or schedule where routine and sustained practice are likely to succeed?

4. Are you willing, when you are faced with a challenge, to see yourself beyond that challenge, visualize it, and actually "feel" the physiological state of being beyond that challenge?

The next metaphor that is appropriate in our transformative process is that of a garden. In *Nowhere Else: Wisdom for Daily Life*, Yves Bertrand talks about the strange psychological powers of a garden.[2] I would liken a garden to the center of the internal self. Bertrand claims that through the strange psychological powers of a garden, stressed individuals who enter become progressively calmer as they advance further into its depths. The further they penetrate a garden and discover its different aspects, the more their demeanor changes.

Now at the center of our labyrinth, we have examined physiological techniques designed for deep internal change, higher emotional states from which to function, and higher states of consciousness. We have also examined the tough questions of true willingness. Before we begin the journey outward, we must look at the readiness of change and steps we can take to facilitate that change. "Tilling the soil" and "our energy diet" are considerations appropriate for our garden metaphor. These terms refer to those practices that can better ready us for change. These external activities that help reduce the stress and chaos in our lives, so we can be better grounded in an internally coherent state, are presented in Chapter Ten.

The Questions of Willingness
EXERCISE AND REFLECTION #9

Reread the questions of willingness presented in this chapter. Process and reflect on specific areas of willingness in your own life, and address the appropriate questions in a way that is meaningful for you. Address the general questions of willingness as well as the questions regarding willingness of practice.

_____

_____

_____

_____

_____

_____

_____

_____

_____

_____

_____

Dimensions of Wellness
ACTIVITY AND REFLECTION #10

Part of being willing to change is allowing ourselves to focus on and appreciate our strengths. The term *wholistic* (or *holistic,* as it is spelled in most circles) is used to represent the idea that we are whole human beings. To authentically engage in living a "well" life, we must consider our whole person, not just our physical health. In the field of wellness, it is well accepted that different aspects or dimensions of health comprise our lives. Although some of these dimensions may be different according to the source representing them, the idea is that we need to pay attention to all of these areas to live a genuinely whole and balanced life. A life out of balance is a life prone to chaos.

It seems to be the nature of our culture to be more comfortable focusing on lack or what is deficient rather than what is positive or abundant. A theme underlying many discussions throughout this book is that if we can shift our constant emotional focus to appreciation, gratitude, love, and compassion, for ourselves as well as for others, profound changes happen in our lives. These changes come from the fact that the attention we hold, in every moment of every day, creates the brain patterns and perceptions by which we live.

It is hard for most of us to sincerely and lovingly, without arrogance or self-importance, allow ourselves to focus on our strengths. Additionally, when we come from a loving or appreciative state when dealing with an issue or aspect of our lives we would like to develop, positive perceptions of change are more abundant.

Following are the identified dimensions of wellness for our purposes, along with a short description of each. Carefully follow the directions as you answer the following:

1. Sit in a comfortable chair where your diaphragm has room to move and take a few deep, slow, and comfortable breaths.

2. As you continue to breathe slowly, deeply, and comfortably, consciously release all the tension around your eyes.

3. Keep your attention on your breath and consciously release the tension in your shoulders. Silently repeat the word "release" on the out breath.

4. Bring your attention to an area in your chest that may be comfortable for you—your solar plexus, heart, "gut," or the area of your lungs as if you're breathing straight through your chest (this helps turn off the chatter in your brain).

5. Generate a strong sense of gratitude for yourself and your strengths. Let yourself genuinely feel a sense of grateful acceptance for your innermost strengths and let this acceptance engulf your body for a few minutes while you continue to breathe.

6. For each identified area, focus on and write about your strengths. After you have authentically shared your strengths, if it is appropriate, identify areas you would like to improve.

Spiritual, but not necessarily religious; the innermost aspect of who you are:

_____

_____

_____

_____

_____

_____

Physical, including your physical capabilities and health:

_____

_____

_____

_____

_____

_____

Social (interpersonal relationships that support who you are at a deep level):

_____

_____

_____

_____

_____

_____

_____

Intellectual (the time you devote to developing your intellect):

_____

_____

_____

_____

_____

_____

Emotional, including both your reaction patterns and where you keep your "feeling" attention:

_____

_____

_____

_____

_____

_____

How did you feel when writing about your strengths? Was it easy to do? What strengths are most important to you? (These may not necessarily be your greatest strengths.) How can you incorporate your most deeply felt strengths into more of your life? Reflect and process in a way that is meaningful to you.

_____

_____

_____

_____

_____

_____

_____

REFERENCES

1. Astin, A. W., and J. P. Keen, "Equanimity and Spirituality," *Religion and Education* 33:2(2006): 1–8.

2. Bertrand, Yves. *Nowhere Else: Wisdom for Daily Life.* Madison, WI: Atwood Publishing, 2004.

Tilling the Soil

Creating Optimal Conditions for Growth

In the first part of this book, I presented the science and physiology of how and why internal experience basically creates who we are. Beyond being personally fascinated by the science, I believe its explanation is necessary to give validity to the concept that where we keep our attention every moment of every day profoundly determines who we become. Additionally, the science proves and supports the idea that intentionally cultivating higher emotional states from which to operate from, profoundly affects not only our external environment, but who we are internally, down to the level of our cells. Finally, I believe that intentionally cultivating higher emotional states will not only lead us to higher potential, higher levels of empowerment, and a higher functioning level of happiness, but it will also lead us to higher levels of consciousness.

The focus of the second part of this book so far has been on the innermost aspect of internal experience, and in our labyrinth metaphor, that focus has brought us to the very center. When you walk a labyrinth, you usually pause in the center and reflect on what you have learned from the journey inward. The experience of moving inward to the labyrinth's center often changes the people who take that journey. The techniques presented for higher emotional refocusing represent the core of our internal experience. Making an intentional and routine shift to higher emotional states changes who we are at the core. We have seen the evidence of this change at the level of our cells, our bodies, our brains, and our psyches.

Still entertaining the innermost aspect of internal experience, we addressed the questions of willingness and allowance. Are you really willing and ready to choose a different internal experience? Will you permit or allow yourself to function differently, with some concrete examples of how to do so? After pausing in the middle of a labyrinth, you begin to journey out. However, the goal of the journey out is to bring what you have learned from the journey inward out into the functioning world.

From our journey inward we have learned, down to a scientific level, the utmost importance of internal experience. Pausing in the center we have learned some specific techniques to transform negative reactive internal experience to positive internal experience. We have learned the fundamental requirement of action in the change process—in this case, the routine and consistent focus on higher states—and we have entertained willingness. Now we begin the journey outward. Now we begin to examine how the intentional cultivation of external experience and circumstance enhances our inner development.

At this point the metaphor or symbol of a pebble in a still pond is fitting. When the pebble first hits the pond, all the ensuing ripples reverberate out from the initial point of contact, with that point being the most important for the effects that follow. I make this point because many programs or philosophies aimed at personal growth begin with manipulating the external experience expecting the internal to follow. In other words, they are based on the concept that if one can change the external environment or circumstance, the internal change will necessarily follow. Even some of the current programs based on attraction or intention seem to focus more on the external gain rather than initially beginning with the internal experience. While both of these approaches may be effective in creating some level of internal change, I deeply believe that to see profound and lasting change we must start at the very center; we must start where the pebble comes in contact with the pond.

After the pebble hits the water, the ripples begin to reverberate out. It is at this point that we need to consider external circumstance as it relates to internal experience. The focus of the rest of this book is on creating external circumstance so that it is conducive to positive internal experience, or higher states of being, fully cognizant of the science behind those higher states of being. We begin initially with what I call "tilling the soil."

A garden, at its deepest sense, is a place of growth. It is a place of dedication, where the miracles of life and growth are acknowledged. For a garden to flourish, first it must be given the conditions of optimal growth. The weeds and the rocks must be removed; the soil must be prepared to sustain the growth that is to take place.

In the same way, as we begin our journey outward, we need to look at the optimal conditions for our own growth. As the book progresses and culminates, we will look at larger issues of external circumstance; however, at this stage we need to focus on creating an environment that can encourage and sustain change. Several of the topics that will be examined may, on the surface, not look like topics addressing the cultivation of internal experience. However, I encourage you to look at these topics in a new light. As the soil of a garden needs to be prepared to be ripe for planting and ultimately affects the potential success for growth, so do we need to create the internal and external practices conducive to growth.

Although these practices will be different for each of us, and you will be asked to reflect on your own personal considerations at the end of the chapter, a few practices are somewhat universally accepted. These are exercise, diet, simplicity, and meditation. After we take a closer look at these four aspects of internal experience, or "tilling the soil," we will examine in Chapter Eleven our own personal "energy diet," or those things that we expose ourselves to on a daily basis that profoundly affect our internal experience.

As was stated early on in the process of this book, stress, chaos, and anxiety cut us off from clear, coherent, and higher levels of internal experience. Additionally, we can undertake specific practices to better ready or prepare ourselves for personal growth. I encourage you to look at these practices in a new light. Beyond the external benefits of these practices, the internal benefits are even greater.

These four practices seem to be the most widely promoted in terms of personal growth; they are also the most important for me personally. These activities and practices can be viewed on a continuum of their potential benefits depending on your comfort level with the idea of intentionally cultivating higher internal experience. At the very least and of fundamental importance are their phenomenal capabilities of reducing the stress, chaos, and anxiety from our lives. There are very real, very measurable, physical and psychological benefits to these practices.

These practices are so important in my own life I often declare that they are what keeps me balanced and in tune with who I am at my deepest level. I find it hard to function without attention paid to each one of these areas, and I can honestly say that each area has profoundly changed my life. Numerous books have been written on each of these topics; however, for our purposes and need for brevity, we will only entertain a belief overview and specifics of how to effectively incorporate each area into your life.

Exercise

What does exercise have to do with internal experience? My friend John from the coffee shop, who is a retired pastor, says plainly, "I'm a nicer person when I exercise." I have another friend who says nothing is more influential on how he will feel psychologically on any given day than the way he feels physically.

Most of us are so desensitized to the recommendation of exercise that we either already do it or just ignore the recommendation when it comes up. Exercise has been shown to be responsible for almost immeasurable health benefits, yet the majority of Americans remain inactive. Exercise is most often seen as the way to a good-looking and fit body, with secondary health benefits. After more than 25 years of experience in health promotion, I can honestly say that most people I have seen beginning to engage in exercise (this figure is literally more than 20,000) have done so for the desired changes in their physique. However, those people who have adopted it as their lifestyle have maintained it mostly for internal reasons, including self-concept, self-esteem, self-acceptance, and feelings of internal peace.

I encourage you to look at exercise in a new light. Although all the external changes in physique will certainly come, along with all the touted and important health benefits, the benefits from reduced stress, chaos, and anxiety, as well as increased self-esteem, self-concept and internal coherence, cannot be understated. Routine cardiorespiratory exercise cuts down on the negative hormones and biochemicals produced by and associated with stress. This type of exercise can increase the endorphins associated with clearer and more coherent thinking, and a body that functions more optimally houses an intellect, a soul, and a spirit that function more optimally. The body truly is the temple of the soul; I have personally seen consistent exercise transform many people's lives.

As volumes can be and are written on the benefits of and ways to partake in exercise, we will take only a brief look at the types of exercise most conducive to creating positive internal experience and concrete ways to develop the habit. Again, as in other behavior change practices, unless you can progress from "knowledge about" (the contemplation phase) to "practice of" (the action phase), there will be no change in behavior—just a very knowledgeable "contemplator." I can honestly say that exercise is an absolute integral part of my life and I feel cut off from the most internal parts of who I am when I don't exercise. We need to be able to cut through the static of life to hear and get in touch with our internal selves. Exercise helps cut through that static.

Components of Fitness

The American College of Sports Medicine (ACSM), the most accepted governing body of sports and fitness, has defined five components of fitness: (1) cardiorespiratory fitness, or exercise designed to keep your heart, lungs, and circulatory system healthy; (2) muscular strength; (3) muscular endurance; (4) flexibility; and (5) body composition. All of these areas are important to overall fitness, and which ones you focus on are a matter of personal choice. However, it is important to know how each component benefits health to decide which is most appropriate for you. I call this the *roadmap to fitness* because without this knowledge, it is like getting into a car at point A and expecting to make it to point B with no clear directions of how to get there. Again, this is all presented in the context of internal experience; however, how we feel and how we feel about ourselves is such an integral part of that experience that fitness gains can have a big impact.

Muscular strength is achieved by resistance exercise (usually weight training) and is more often associated with shaping, building, and strengthening muscle mass. **Muscular endurance** is achieved by resistance exercise with lighter weights than muscular strength requires; it can also be done by resistance of body weight or another apparatus designed for resistance. Muscular endurance focuses more on the repetitive movement of the muscle, and although muscular strength usually requires heavier weight at lesser repetitions—about 75 percent 1 RM, or repetition max, the measurement of the most weight you can do in one repetition of a specific exercise—muscular endurance increase requires sets of about eight to fifteen reps at about 50 percent 1 RM.

Muscular strength and endurance are the exercises most responsible for muscle and body sculpting and, to a much lesser extent, body fat loss. When you work on resistance exercise, especially muscular strength, you should not work the same muscle group on consecutive days, as you are actually causing micro-tears in the muscle tissue and need to give that tissue a chance to heal. That's how the muscle gets stronger.

Flexibility gains are specific to the joint stretched. Flexibility and resistance exercise are both important to trunk strength, proper body alignment, and the overall health of the musculoskeletal system. To get a clearer picture of the musculoskeletal system, imagine a pile of sticks held in upright formation by a whole system of rubber bands. This is how the skeletal and muscular systems work together to become the musculoskeletal system. Balance of the opposing muscles in this system is extremely important for those bones (or sticks in our analogy) to be held in place and function properly. This balance is achieved through proper development in opposing muscle groups through resistance exercise as well as attention to flexibility.

Cardiorespiratory endurance gains require sustained, rhythmic, and continuous exercise, although lesser health gains can certainly be achieved by keeping moderately active with various other activities that require the body to move. I always use as a rule of thumb that the more and bigger the muscles you engage in the activity, the more the fitness gains. By sustained continuous exercise I mean brisk walking, jogging, swimming, cycling, aerobics, many types of conditioning equipment designed for those types of fitness gains, and sports with a continuous movement component like soccer or basketball.

Body composition is the makeup of the body in terms of the ratio of body fat as opposed to other types of tissue, including muscle and internal organs. Changes in body composition also require sustained, continuous, and rhythmic exercise, but more of it. To really see significant changes in body composition, the ACSM recommends that you do this type of exercise for thirty to sixty minutes at least five days a week. You can measure this type of activity by the metabolic cost, or calories burned. Simply put, to lose a significant amount of body fat, you need to burn enough calories.

Planning for Success

Exercise for cardiorespiratory endurance and body composition changes, or what we sometimes call *aerobic exercise*, is also the type of exercise most associated with stress reduction. It is most associated with stress reduction because of the biochemical changes that it produces. These biochemical changes counteract the biochemical damage that occurs as a result of stress. Additionally, because body image is often associated with self-esteem, and low self-esteem and self-concept greatly reduce positive internal experience, in my opinion this type of exercise is most closely associated with enhancing and developing positive, or higher internal experience. For me, there's no question. I'm much more connected with who I am at my deepest levels when I routinely exercise. I'm much less reactive, more internally focused and directed, and much happier, clear, and coherent existing in my own body.

How does all this information transfer into a higher internal experience? By actually doing it. From behavior change and fitness research, we know exercise needs to be put into action to be effective. We also know that certain conditions make it more likely to become action. If you don't like or enjoy what you are doing, you probably won't stick to it. My first and foremost recommendation is to find something you like and make it FUN. Yes, make it fun. Find a group of people to do it with, listen to music, move in a way that feels good, but make sure you enjoy it.

My second recommendation is to build it into your daily schedule. If it's not built in to your daily schedule, it will always fall victim to other things on your agenda. Third, create a social support system. This social support system could be a group of people to do it with, it could be a system of people that support you to get it done by yourself. You know the type of support that would be most beneficial for you. Think about it ahead of time and create this network to help you move from contemplation to action. The fourth and fifth recommendations are to record your progress and prepare for "accidentally quitting."

Accidentally quitting is when something happens, some legitimate reason why you need to take a break, but that break becomes a week, and then two weeks, etc. Pretty soon you've quit the routine without ever intending to do so. How do you recognize when this has happened? How do you get yourself back on track? It could be as simple as a phone call from a friend, watching an inspirational movie, or whatever you have put in place to remind yourself of this phenomenon. Being able to recognize it, understanding that it happens all the time, and getting yourself back on track are the keys to not letting an accidental respite from your routine become permanent.

The Importance of Exercise
EXERCISE AND REFLECTION #11

What types of exercise do you think would best contribute to a higher internal experience? Why? What exactly would you do?

_____

_____

_____

_____

_____

_____

What specifically would be the best way to incorporate this or these activities into your life? Who? What? Where? When? How? Be specific.

_____

_____

_____

_____

_____

_____

What would be the best way for you to get back on track after "accidentally quitting"? How would you carry this through?

_____

_____

_____

_____

_____

Process and reflect on concrete ways you can move from contemplation to action and sincerely engage in and make these activities a routine part of your life.

_____

_____

_____

_____

_____

_____

Meditation or Mental Practice

There is absolutely no other activity that I believe leads to higher potential, higher internal development, and higher states of consciousness than meditation. A large part of this book has been devoted to the internal and physiological benefits of activities similar to meditation or other internal practices. Because there are many different types and forms of meditation and because covering all of those types would be far beyond the scope of this book, I direct you back to the sustained practice of the higher emotional and refocusing techniques presented in Chapters Seven and Eight.

Again these techniques were developed for ease of use and in no way claim superiority over other techniques. However, they are designed to be simple, adaptable for use anytime, anywhere, and useful for everyone, regardless of experience in mental or emotional training techniques. The most important aspect is moving from contemplation to action; it is in actually performing, routinely and consistently, the activity that will bring about change. This book is full of the scientific and physiological rationale why these types of practices induce change, but that change will not happen if you don't engage in the practices sincerely and routinely.

If you are interested in other types of meditative practices, I encourage you to explore various techniques and find what feels comfortable and natural for you. There are numerous books on all types of meditation, as well as general books on meditative practice. My personal library is full of these books, and the best recommendation I can make is to find a practice that resonates with you.

I encourage you to develop your own practice, one that feels most comfortable for you based on all the available resources. Remember all the foundational and physiological changes that can happen with routine practice; these changes are more likely to happen with a practice that feels comfortable for you, and one that you are most likely to engage in routinely. Meditation, like exercise, will be a much more successful practice if it is something that you truly enjoy doing and from which you feel personal benefit. There are many traditions and suggestions for developing a practice that works for you; I encourage you to explore and find a practice in which you will routinely, consistently, and sincerely engage.

Additionally, as in exercise, social support can be a wonderful asset in developing a sustained practice. Many organized groups routinely meet and practice numerous types of meditation, some even at colleges and universities. Furthermore, the group atmosphere is wonderfully conducive to getting the most benefit and encouraging routine practice. Even if you have established your own personal sustained practice, occasional group practice can be a great asset, in that group practice can bring the whole experience to a higher level.

Also, as in exercise, sustained meditative practice is much more likely to be successful and carried out routinely if you have a specific place and schedule to do so. Again, it is the routine experience that creates the changes, and paying attention and creating circumstances conducive to practice are necessary steps to ensuring consistency. Do what you need to do to move your practice or thoughts of practice from contemplation to action.

Sustained Meditation Practice
EXERCISE AND REFLECTION #12

Reread the section on sustained HEART in Chapter Eight. Reflect and process whether this type of practice or another routine meditative practice is something you would like to develop. Why or why not? If another type of practice is attractive to you, is there a specific one that appeals to you? What are the aspects that attract you most to this type of practice, and what would be the necessary conditions for you to create in your life to maintain a successful practice? The benefits of this type of practice cannot be overstated. Routine and consistent practice changes us at the cellular level, at the neural level, and all of our behaviors, perceptions, and actions follow from there. Reflect and process whether it is appropriate for you and how you can incorporate some form of sustained practice into your daily life. Be specific, be creative, and do what works for you.

_____

_____

_____

_____

_____

_____

_____

_____

_____

_____

Simplicity

One of the main messages of this book is that we need to cut through the stress, chaos, and anxiety in our lives to be able to access our internal selves and create calm, productive, and positive internal experience. From this internal experience, the rest of our existence develops. Voluntary simplicity, not simplicity forced from lack of necessary and fundamental necessities, is an important aspect of this process. Quite often we create and live our lives flooded with the countless demands of overconsumption, overscheduling, and an over-driven mentality that we have no idea how to get in touch with our internal selves, or even that we have such a thing as an internal self.

As I mentioned in Chapter One, most people view stress management as a method of merely controlling the chaos and scheduling the chaos so it is "workable" rather than sub-stantially reducing it from our lives. Looking inward helps us reduce that chaos, and volun-tary simplicity helps us to look inward. If our lives are full of the demands of an over-the-top lifestyle, we don't have the time, attention, or energy to be able to give to our internal experience. How can you listen to the voice of your internal self if you can't even hear it because it is either cluttered physically or psychologically with too much of everything?

Voluntary simplicity means we make conscious choices to reduce our overconsump-tion, our cluttered environments, our overly burdensome workloads, and our constant tech-nological overstimulation. We make a concerted effort to balance our inner and outer development. This is a complete paradigm shift from the mentality that more is better and if we accumulate enough possessions or enough external validation, somehow we will feel better about ourselves. Its like my friend Violet Scolinos said, "It seems like our culture is on this frantic treadmill and we're afraid to get off, because if we do we'll have to look inside ourselves." Voluntary simplicity helps us slow this treadmill down. Voluntary sim-plicity helps us see the roses so that we can actually stop and smell them.

What does voluntary simplicity mean in concrete terms? This answer is as individual as we are. I believe we all, at some intuitive level, know what the answers are for us. Are you a "pack rat"? Do you impulsively shop thinking that some thing or acquisition will make you feel better somehow? Are you constantly overstimulated with technology, includ-ing computers, cell phones, TV, and video games? Does it take more time and effort to take care of your acquisitions than the enjoyment you derive from them? Have you over-loaded your life with so many commitments that you overlook time for yourself, to be silent or spend in nature? Do you always have to be busy? Do you know how to say "no" when it is appropriate? What is it that you feel especially overwhelmed by, and how can you take steps to simplify the conditions surrounding that feeling of being overwhelmed?

I have made a concerted effort to reduce many of these complications in my own life, but simplifying my physical environment seems to be a constant battle. With two teenage boys, two big dogs, and two cats as well as working full time and being a passionate author, keeping my physical environment simple is a challenge. However, I have come to realize its importance. As with exercise, diet, and meditation, if my physical environment is out of my comfort zone, I just feel bad.

Part of voluntary simplicity is not just reducing the over-the-top behavior, but intentionally cultivating the opposite. When was the last time you chose to be silent and felt comfortable in that silence? When was the last time you walked in the woods or on the beach? When was the last time you looked at the stars? When was the last time you decided to go a day or week with no computer, cell phone, or TV? When was the last time you decided to forgo buying something because you really didn't need it or probably wouldn't use it anyway? When is the last time you decided to clear the clutter and throw out everything you haven't used in the past year?

Voluntary simplicity is as individual as we each are and these are just a few recommendations to consider. What I recommend at a much deeper level is for you to honestly examine areas in your life that could benefit from intentional simplification. Again, it's like the metaphor of the statue of David. It is said that when Michelangelo sculpted David, he removed all the parts that weren't David and David began to appear. What keeps you from time, effort, and energy to devote to internal higher cultivation?

Voluntary Simplification
EXERCISE AND REFLECTION #13

Process and reflect on the information presented in the previous section. What resonates with you? Where in your life do you feel overwhelmed? Do you take time for your inner development? What prevents you from doing so? Read over all the questions presented in this section, ask yourself any other questions that may be appropriate, and reflect how you can intentionally create more simplicity in your life.

_____

_____

_____

_____

_____

_____

_____

_____

_____

_____

_____

Diet

Few things allow me a more positive or negative internal experience than the nutrition I give to my body. We are holistic beings. It is often said that the body is the temple of the soul. The paradox is I truly believe we are internal beings with a physical body, but how well we take care of that physical body determines, to a great extent, our level of internal experience. Simply put, how we feel physically and how we feel about our physical bodies has a great impact on how we feel internally. What is more, the nutrition and fuel we give to our bodies greatly determines how we physically feel.

Consequently, how do we create a nurturing and health-promoting diet for ourselves with the onslaught of information and misinformation available in our current culture? One of the benefits of spending so many years in the health promotion profession is being able to critically examine the numerous trends and fads I have seen come and go. Nowhere is that more apparent than in the field of diet and nutrition. I use the term *nutrition* lightly in connection with these fads because some of the diet trends that have been popular in the last thirty years bear little resemblance to anything nutritionally sound.

If you take a brief look at all the nutritional trends embraced by American popular culture in the last three decades, you see drastically different recommendations, but each during its time was regarded as *the* answer. We went from extremely low carbohydrates, to almost no fat, to diet shakes, to low protein, to high protein, and back to extremely low carbohydrates. There have been numerous miracle supplements along the way that promised to make you lose weight while you slept or to mimic the results of exercise so you effectively got the benefits of exercise straight from the bottle. There were supplements that promised to block the absorption of carbohydrates, so you could eat as much as you wanted without absorbing the calories; supplements that claimed to be "fat blockers"; and numerous supplements that promised to speed up your metabolism. Unfortunately, this final claim was accomplished by speeding up the muscle called your heart and thinning your blood, which unfortunately could be fatal.

Many food labels are so deceptive in their claims they might as well be outright lies, and the diet and food supplement industry continues to grow at astronomical proportions. Our culture is bombarded with all these miracle diets and miracle products, yet obesity has now surpassed smoking as the leading cause of preventable death in the United States. Why? In my opinion it is because we have been looking in the wrong place. When we make the shift to looking at food and nutrition as fuel for our souls rather than something we need to do to maintain society's ideal of the perfect external body, we can begin to let go of the absurd emotional dependence we have created for ourselves.

When we exhibit negative reactive patterns and negative self-talk associated with body image, body type, or health concerns regarding diet, those negative reactive patterns create the circumstance conducive to failure. All at once we are drawn to the latest diet fad, yet we find ourselves eating fast food, junk food, and food that is not healthy for our own specific nutritional needs. As has been the focus of much of this book, I believe that the best way to adopt a lifestyle or personal pattern that is conducive to internal development is to replace the negative pattern with a positive one rather than just trying to get rid of the negative.

How does this work when it comes to nutrition? Look inward. Feed your body, feed your soul. Create a positive nurturing experience, an attitude that your body, brain, and reactive patterns will follow suit and where the focus is on the positive emotional development of giving your body the nutrition it needs. Your body will naturally gravitate to healthy, fresh, and nutrient-dense food. You will automatically crave what your body needs.

Additionally, remember our discussion on biochemistry and oxytocin. If you are creating enough positive loving and nurturing practices, both internally by intentional practice and externally by creating loving connections with yourself and those around you, you won't need to fill the void biochemically by faulty eating.

How does this all work in actual practice? In the next several pages you will be asked to do various activities, and you will be presented with a basic overview of nutrition. Through the completion of these activities, you will be able to create a sound nutritional plan for yourself. This plan will support a positive and loving internal experience that cuts through the chaos and negative emotionalism created by an industry that profits when you fail.

The first activity directs you to pay careful attention to how the nutrients you give your body serve you in an internal sense, or how you feel after ingesting them. Then, with a better understanding of the nutrients or food sources that personally serve you, the next step is to examine basics of nutrition and variations that may or may not be appropriate for you. After you are armed with this information, you will be led through the process of creating an individual nutrition plan based on your individual needs, preferences, and any desires you may have for physical change.

Daily Food and Response Log
EXERCISE AND REFLECTION #14

Everybody's body is different. The ways different people respond to various nutrients are vast, and no one diet or nutritional plan is appropriate for everyone. This activity is designed to help you become aware of which foods serve you and which do not. It is designed to provide a gauge for eating behaviors that may or may not be conducive to positive internal experience or merely feeling good. For at least four days, record everything you ingest. This is meant to be a log of your typical behavior, not a record of four days where you intentionally manipulate your diet. Include everything you ingest, including medications and liquids (alcohol, water, coffee, etc.). The more honest you can be, the more this process will provide useful information.

This activity is not about diet analysis, but about reflecting and processing on how your personal habits are serving you. Record everything you ingest, how you felt an hour later, how you felt three to four hours later, and any comments about what you ate and its connection to how you felt. Under the comments, also record how much sleep you had the previous evening and what activities you engaged in that may have affected your energy level. These activities and their effect on how you feel physically will vary greatly. Sitting, reading, and writing can be as draining sometimes as physical activity. The key for this whole exercise is to make it as individual as you can about your eating, sleeping, and activity behaviors in the moment, within a few hours, and even the next day.

How did you feel when you woke up?	Time and food eaten	How you felt one hour later	How you felt three hours later	Sleep, activities, and further comments

How did you feel when you woke up?	Time and food eaten	How you felt one hour later	How you felt three hours later	Sleep, activities, and further comments

Process and Reflect

How did you feel physically throughout this process? Does anything stand out as valuable information? How did you feel internally? How did you feel physically and internally when you woke up each day? Can you relate that feeling to what you consumed the day before? Was your energy level optimal?

_____

_____

_____

_____

_____

_____

_____

_____

_____

_____

_____

_____

Your personal habits are profoundly intertwined with the physiological process presented in this book. Your personal habits profoundly affect your internal experience of life, and any repeated internal experience creates and strengthens biochemical reaction patterns, neural networks, perceptions, and behaviors. Paying attention to how your personal habits make you feel is the first step in having this process work for you and help you make positive changes in your life rather than the opposite.

Nutrition Basics

Foods are basically made up of three components—carbohydrates, fats, and proteins—and knowledge about each and their function will help you decide how much of each and what sources are best for you individually. Additionally, other components of food or food types are included because of their importance or common inclusion in our diet. Those are fiber, fruits, vegetables, and alcohol.

Carbohydrates

Carbohydrates are comprised of sugars and starches, which are broken down into glucose in your body and used for energy. The general category of carbohydrates is broken down into subcategories of complex and simple, as determined by the complexity of their chemical structure and how fast they are broken down and converted into sugar by your body. Carbohydrates can be "good" or "bad" depending on their density of nutrients, their level of complexity, and your personal sensitivity to their consumption. Typically, a more active person needs a higher carbohydrate diet, and a less active person needs a lower carbohydrate diet. Additionally, if you have medical problems involving blood sugar, you should rely on much more complex carbohydrates and a lower carbohydrate diet overall. The USDA recommends that about 50 to 70 percent of your daily caloric needs be met by carbohydrates. Each gram of carbohydrate has four calories.

Fats

Fats are also used as an energy source. They are a much more concentrated energy source and one that is slower in availability to the body. A fat can also be classified as "good" or "bad" depending on whether it is saturated and whether its chemical structure has been altered, as in trans-fatty acids. Research in recent years has shown trans-fatty acids to be the most unhealthy of all fats. The USDA recommends that an adult diet include include 20 to 35 percent fats, with no more than 10 percent from the saturated or trans-fatty acids category. Each gram of fat has nine calories.

Proteins

Proteins are the building blocks of life. They are made up of amino acids and are primarily responsible for many body processes. They form the basis for all cells. The body goes through a complicated process to convert them to energy, so they are generally not used for energy, except in cases where carbohydrates and fats are not available. The USDA recommends that the diet be comprised of 10 to15 percent protein; however, intake in a high protein diet may be up to 30 percent. It is important to note that when a diet is this high in protein, it is also usually low in carbohydrates, meaning that fats make up the difference. If you are on a high protein/low carbohydrate diet, it is extremely important to make sure the higher level of fat is obtained through healthy sources. A gram of protein yields four calories.

Fiber

Fiber is an important component in our diets for overall health. It is a carbohydrate that cannot be digested. Higher levels of fiber help with digestion, help lower blood sugar, and help lower cholesterol. Fiber is found most densely in whole grains, fruits, and vegetables. The USDA daily recommendation is approximately 25 grams for women and 38 grams for men. Most of us do not come close to meeting this requirement.

Fruits and Vegetables

I personally believe that fruits and vegetables are the powerhouse of any healthy diet, especially one directed at creating a higher internal experience. Fruits and vegetables are nutrient dense and, for the most part, calorically sparse. They contain antioxidants, fiber, water, vitamins, and minerals and thus should be the foundation of a person's diet. Added to other foods, they can provide bulk and reduce overall caloric content of a meal without reducing volume.

Alcohol

With seven calories to a gram, alcohol is a concentrated and empty source of calories. In other words, it usually provides an ample source of calories but no positive nutrients. Some health benefits have been associated with moderate consumption of alcohol, especially red wine. Unless there is a personal or familial history of alcoholism, blood sugar issues, or other health problems, moderate consumption of alcohol appears to have no overt negative effects. Moderate amounts of alcohol are defined as no more than one drink per day for women and no more than two drinks per day for men. A drink is defined as five ounces of wine, one ounce of liquor, or one 12-ounce beer. The differing amounts for men and women are because women are generally smaller and metabolize alcohol at a slower rate. Additionally, the recommendations for women may be lower if there is a personal or familial history of breast cancer.

Putting It Together

How do you take all this information, individualize it, and put it in a usable format? Remember moving from contemplation to action is the most important step in behavior change. Taking action in proper nutrition starts with a specific and individualized plan.

First of all, a calorie is a measurement of energy that a specific food gives you. Body fat is merely stored energy. The energy balance equation tells us that if we take more energy in than we expend, we store that energy in the form of body fat. If we expend more energy than we consume, we access the stored energy in body fat. If our goal is to remain the same weight, we balance energy in (calories) with energy out (basic life functions and exercise). Contrary to some claims, calories do count in the energy balance equation.

We can figure out what we need in the way of carbohydrates, protein, and fats based on a specific and individualized caloric intake. We can learn to read food labels, reflect on what foods make us feel healthy, and create an optimal nutrition plan for ourselves. Additionally, if our desire is to lose or gain weight, we can manipulate the caloric allowance up or down, add exercise, and create a plan with these goals in mind.

The first step is to identify caloric needs. Following are general recommendations. Everybody is different, and these recommendations are for a person of average size and healthy weight, with minimal activity. If you would like more specific guidelines, I encourage you to visit http://www.mpyramid.gov. This web site offers in-depth and valuable information for many dietary and health concerns.

Caloric Requirements

Most women and girls	1,800
Women over 60	1,600
Active women	2,000
Inactive boys and men	2,200
Active boys and men	2,500

Judge for yourself where you need to be, and adjust up or down to a level that feels right depending on your personal metabolism. Additionally, if you want to lose or gain weight, don't count the activity yet. In other words, if I am an active female, but I still want to lose weight, at this point I would count the caloric requirement established for an inactive female, so I can use the calories allotted for activity in the following weight loss formula.

Enter your estimated recommended calories on the activity sheet following this section. The following recommendations are to be followed if you desire to lose or gain weight. A pound of body fat is equal to 3,500 calories. In other words, it takes a 3,500 caloric deficit to lose a pound of body fat. The most effective way to do this is combine a caloric deficit through reducing food intake and increasing activity level. If you are trying to gain weight, you would aim to create a caloric surplus through intake. Because 3,500 calories is equal to a pound, and the safest, most effective way to lose and keep weight off is to lose one or two pounds a week, you would combine the calories used during exercise with a deficit created from a reduction in food intake to amount to somewhere between 3,500 and 7,000 calories a week, or 500 to 1,000 a day.

Cardiorespiratory or aerobic exercise is most effective in burning a substantial amount of calories. How many calories burned depends on body size, intensity of exercise, duration of exercise, and the activity you do. Generally, jogging about a ten-minute mile burns about 100 calories; and if you can compare your activity to that equation and adjust it up or down accordingly, you will have a good estimation.

Remember, you can only subtract the exercise calories for the days you are actually performing the exercise. If you are trying to reduce your body fat, subtract your exercise calories from the needed deficit and you will have an adjusted deficit. This adjusted deficit needs to be subtracted from your original recommended daily calories.

For example, the recommended caloric needs for an adult female are 1,800, but a woman nearing 50 with a slower metabolism might find 1,600 to be more appropriate. If this woman wants to lose 1½ pounds a week, she would need to trim 750 calories from her daily intake or burn some or all of those calories through additional exercise. She runs four miles a day, fast enough to burn about 400 calories. So, she can subtract 400 from 750, meaning that she now needs to trim 350 calories from her daily intake, which brings her new adjusted recommendation to 1,250 calories. This is in a safe range, as the American College of Sports Medicine recommends that daily caloric intake not be lower than 1,200.

Whether you want to maintain, lose, or gain weight, you should have a recommended caloric intake for each day. If you want to maintain your current weight, you can find your recommended caloric intake in the answer to question 1 on the following exercise. If you want to gain or lose weight, look to the answer to question 7. Now refer back to the nutrition basics, guidelines, and importance of carbohydrates, fats, and proteins. Then review your daily food log and examine if any particular type of food seems especially beneficial or detrimental for you. Take this into account in your examination of the role fats, proteins, and carbohydrates do and should play for you. On question 8, estimate, within the recommended range, where you should fall for each of the food sources. If you are more active and seem to function better on higher carbohydrates, list a number closer to 70 percent. If you are less active and are especially sensitive to blood sugar issues, list a lower number. Do this as well for fats and proteins.

For question 9, take those percentages and multiply them by the recommended amount of daily calories. This number represents the amount of daily calories that should be allotted to carbohydrates, fats, and proteins. Because grams are easier to count, question 10 helps you calculate the amount of grams you need in each area for a balanced and healthy diet.

Food labels clearly state the grams of carbohydrates, fats, and proteins, along with the amount of calories per serving. Pay extra attention to the serving size, which can be surprising. The label often lists a serving size much smaller than what people typically consume, so the actual intake of fats, carbohydrates, protein, and calories consumed is higher than the label states.

For foods that are fresh and not in a labeled package, which I recommend comprise a high percentage of your diet, many resources are available in book form and online to provide nutrition information. Some electronic devices are actually programmed so you can enter calories and grams of specific foods and keep track of your daily totals.

Conclusion

Your nutrition plan needs to be individualized and take into account both your personal preferences and the types and amounts of food that are appropriate for your lifestyle and body. You don't need a complicated food plan to create a diet that serves your needs. Eat fresh, healthy, organic fruits and vegetables, if you can get them, and supplement them with healthy fats like nuts, avocados, and healthy oils. Add in some whole grains and lean proteins, and pay attention to how many grams of each food source and total calories you are consuming each day. Avoid processed foods, simple sugars, and refined flours. Use alcohol in moderation, if it's appropriate for you to do so, and pay attention to how what you eat and how much you eat serves you.

Pay attention to how you feel. If you are making a major change in your diet, it may take a few days before you realize the fundamental and foundational benefits of healthy, whole food. Food in our bodies is like gas in a gas tank. Our cars wouldn't run with anything but appropriate fuel sources, yet we expect our bodies to run on less. If you give your body too much or too little food, if you give it toxins and junk, is it any wonder that you feel bad? Your internal experience is profoundly affected by the way you feel physically. The way you feel is profoundly affected by what you put in your body. Pay attention; take good care. Your body is the host of your internal self.

Your Individualized Nutrition Plan
EXERCISE AND REFLECTION #15

Use the information presented on the previous pages to answer the following questions.

1. What do you estimate your daily caloric needs to be? _____

2. Do you want to gain or lose weight? _____ Yes _____ No (if no, go to question 8)

3. If you desire to gain or lose weight, how much per week?

   Circle the caloric deficit required for that amount. (If you want to gain weight, go to question 7.)

   1 lb _____ = 500 cal/day

   1½ lbs _____ = 750 cal/day

   2 lbs _____ = 1,000 cal/day

4. If you want to lose weight, will you use aerobic exercise to help? _____ Yes _____ No

5. Estimate how many calories on average you will burn per day: _____

6. If you want to lose weight, subtract the answer of question 5 from the circled value in question 3.

7. If you want to lose weight, subtract the answer to number 6 from the answer to number 1. _____ If you want to gain weight, add the circled number in question 3 to the answer to number 1.

8. a. Estimate the percentage of carbohydrates you need daily _____ (50–70% unless you are on a low carb diet)

   b. Estimate the percentage of fats you need daily _____ (20–35%)

   c. Estimate the percentage of protein you need daily _____ (10–15%)

9. a. Amount of recommended carbohydrate calories multiplied by your total caloric recommendation _____ (#8a × either #1 or #7; #1 if you want to maintain, #7 if you want to lose or gain weight)

   b. Amount of recommended fat calories multiplied by your total caloric recommendation _____ (#8b × either #1 or #7)

   c. Amount of recommended protein calories multiplied by your total caloric recommendation _____ (#8c × either #1 or #7)

10. a. Estimate daily grams of carbohydrates (divide 9a by 4) _____

    b. Estimate daily grams of fat (divide 9b by 9) _____

    c. Estimate daily grams of proteins (divide 9c by 4) _____

Process and Reflect

How can you, considering your current lifestyle, make little or big changes to improve your eating lifestyle? Be specific. How can you take concrete action? Process and brainstorm how you can move from contemplation to action in a way that is appropriate for you.

_____

_____

_____

_____

_____

_____

_____

_____

_____

_____

_____

_____

_____

Our Energy Diet and Subjective Interpretation

The Purpose of an Energy Diet

At this point in our process, it should be absolutely apparent that where we keep our attention every moment of every day, through a complex psycho-physiological process, literally becomes who we are. Everything we expose ourselves to—every thought, every choice, every situation, every relationship—affects our bodies and brains in such a way that determines who we become. Understanding this dynamic gives us the power of choice. Understanding this dynamic gives us the power of manipulation of our surroundings for our good and the good of those around us.

This chapter is built on the concept that the creation of an "energy diet" is foundational in our journey of transformation. By paying careful attention to those things in our lives that may add to or detract from our personal energy, that may, unbeknownst to us, set off a cascade of positive or negative reaction patterns, we can begin to manipulate our surroundings and further our transformative journey.

The term *diet* was chosen as a metaphor for all the things that fuel our existence, everything we ingest in our daily lives. As a nutritional diet is composed of all of the food substances we take in on a daily basis, an energy diet is composed of all of those things that day after day add to or detract from a higher internal experience. Our nutritional diet consists of what we subsist on every day, positive or negative, not just what we eat when we are trying to manipulate our nutritional intake in a positive direction. If we live only on chips and soda, then that is our daily diet, nourishing or not. The same is true of all things in our lives to which we constantly expose ourselves emotionally and physically: our thoughts, our subjective interpretations, our "inner chatter," our surroundings, the things we do, the words we speak, and the people with whom we relate. This chapter invites you to take a deep look at the things in your life that may be contributing to, or detracting from, your ability to develop a higher level of internal experience. Some of these things may be obvious, but others will take some work to uncover. As you delve into these mundane experiences and influences, you may discover some that have a negative impact on your brain and body. Perhaps you will see these aspects of your life in a new light. Uncovering those aspects leads to the power of choice between what is life affirming and what is not and to the power of subjective interpretation, or how you choose to see events or situations.

A persistent message of this book is that every thought or feeling we have creates and strengthens neural networks in our brains and biochemical reaction patterns in our bodies. The stronger these reaction patterns, the more they become ingrained in our way of being. This concept is fundamentally important to consider in what we expose ourselves to every day, in our use of semantics, or the words we choose to use, and in the way we choose to interpret events. The power of semantics will be covered in Chapter Twelve. The focus of this chapter is on what we energetically expose ourselves to by the choices we make and the way we choose to interpret the events of our lives.

External Choices and Internal Experiences

Every time we expose ourselves to something—a thing, situation, thought, or word—that exposure strengthens the neural networks associated with the underlying feeling attached to it. Additionally, every time we have a specific interpretation of an event—and most of the time those interpretations are subjective, or open to any meaning we choose—we strengthen the neural networks associated with those feelings. These neural networks and biochemical reactions profoundly determine our level of internal experience. Furthermore, even if the initial internal experience may seem subtle, repeated experience profoundly determines the overall effect of those choices.

Remember, the level of our internal experience creates more of the same biologically, psychologically, and spiritually in our external lives. The level of our internal experience profoundly affects our perceptions, our behavior, and the choices we make. Our level of internal experience eventually, through all the processes described in this book, determines our baseline level of happiness and how effectively we operate in the world. Our daily choices profoundly affect our internal experiences.

This process happens whether we are aware of it or not. It happens whether we are using it for our benefit or not. To truly grasp this concept, it is important to explore it at a fairly deep level. Many programs or books on self-help or transformation, while their content may be truly powerful, leave out the absolute harm we are doing to ourselves by staying in status quo, by remaining stuck in our current choice behaviors. I believe there is power in knowledge, and understanding the negative impact of many of our subtle, or not so subtle choices, may serve as motivation to change.

What is an energy diet? It consists of everything in our lives that affects us at an implicit or explicit energetic or psychosomatic level. To take charge of our energy diet, we must uncover the things that affect us both at the level of the mind (psycho) and at the level of the body (somatic). Only then can we manipulate those things in a positive way. To put it more simply, we must be able to take note of everything we expose ourselves to, identify whether those things make us "feel good" or "feel bad," and take concrete action to accentuate the positive and reduce the negative.

It is important to remember how we feel psychologically or emotionally about something is directly related to our physiological processes and adaptations—in other words, how our body is adapting and how we feel physically. It is also especially important to pay attention to the subtle, implicit, and previously unnoticed effects that may be going on for us in response to some stimulus. In taking stock of our energy diet, it is important to tune into both how we feel psychologically and how we feel physically in reaction to all aspects of our lives. If something is causing a noticeable physical reaction in us, our bodies have already begun to be invaded by the negative biochemicals and brain synapse patterns associated with the negative reaction to that stimulus. If we want to heal and perform at our optimal level of existence, we must pay attention to this reaction.

Also of fundamental importance in taking stock of our energy diet is the awareness of readiness for change. You may find that some people, places, or things are draining your physical and psychological energy, but for whatever reason you are not ready to take steps for that change. It is important to honor these feelings. Investigate your resistance if you are led to do so, but always honor what is appropriate for you. Taking stock of your energy diet does not require that you live like a monk, unless it is appropriate for you at your current level of development to do so. Taking stock of and improving your energy diet asks you to be deeply aware and mindful of how you feel physically and psychologically in reaction to certain stimuli and to take steps to improve your exposure *where it is appropriate for you to do so*. It also asks you to question some things you may not have questioned in the past.

The Power of Higher Choice

Many current authors address the concept of this type of energetic awareness. Dr. Judith Orloff, in *Positive Energy*, introduces the term "energy vampires" and asks us to be aware of the people in our lives who may be damaging our personal energy.[1] In a personal presentation, Orloff also used the words "on centeredness" to represent the feeling we get when we are paying attention to those things that for us are positive influences in our lives, things that give us an "intuitive yes." Dr. Wayne Dyer, among others, speaks of the concept of vibrational energy and basically asserts that everything we expose ourselves to carries a certain level of energy that is either positive or negative for us.[2]

Dr. David Hawkins has conducted more than thirty years of research in the area of applied kinesiology. This area of study demonstrates the strength or weakness of the body as it is exposed to various stimuli, thoughts, concepts, or ideas. The underlying theory of this research is that our bodies can serve as calibration instruments to assess the vibrational or energetic level of various stimuli.[3] In other words, because of subtle physiological changes we experience when we are exposed to either positive or negative influences, we can actually measure changes in our physical strength.

Whether or not you feel comfortable with the term or concept of vibrational energy, there is no question that every thought, feeling, or emotion we experience creates measurable biochemical, neural, and electrical changes in our bodies. Everything we do, everything we say, everything we expose ourselves to, and every choice we make creates a mind/body connection that literally determines who we become. Sometimes these influences are implicit or subtle, meaning they are only felt subconsciously or minimally; sometimes they are explicit and obvious. The important concept to remember here is that these changes occur as a response to what we expose ourselves to, whether we intentionally manipulate these effects for positive impact or not.

Whether implicit and subtle or explicit and obvious, these situations affect us positively or negatively every minute of every day. Furthermore, just because something may be implicit or subconscious does not mean it is not dramatic in its overall and long-term effect. In other words, if we do not train ourselves to consciously be aware of the negative yet subtle daily influences, choices we make, or words we use, they can have an overall dramatic effect. The challenge is to be aware of how all these situations, thoughts, choices, people, and feelings affect us, to gravitate toward the positive, and to eliminate the negative, as much as it is appropriate for us to do so.

Be kind to and tolerant of yourself in the process. Some will choose to take baby steps; some, with this new awareness, will choose to make more dramatic change. Honor your process. As we noted in Chapter Nine in our discussion of willingness, some people change, or transform, in constant small increments. Others seem to stand still until, with enough inertia, they go through rapid and substantial periods of growth. Honor what is right for you. All the suggestions for transformation in this book are meant to be invitations to implement what resonates with you. Some will take all they can, ready for substantial growth. Some will take a little at a time, implementing what feels comfortable at various times. Some will put the book down, only to pick it up a year from now and deeply go through the process.

What Is Somatic Knowledge?

The term *somatic knowledge* refers to the idea that tuning into our bodies can give us incredibly valuable information about what is healthy for us psychologically, emotionally, and spiritually. In other words, our bodies inherently know what is healthy for us because of the subtle physical changes taking place within them when we are exposed to a thing, a thought, a word, a choice, or an interpretation. Because our bodies are constantly changing in response to what we expose them to, positive and negative, physically and psychologically, tuning into our physical responses serves as sort of a compass for internal or psychological health. It is here we perform and live from our most productive and coherent selves.

The term *internal coherence* has been used quite widely to describe a state when our bodies and minds are functioning at their most optimal, where our biochemical, electrical, and neural patterns are in sync and functioning in a healthy and coherent state. It is here we are most productive, positive, in the "flow," or in the "zone." The objective of creating a positive energy diet is to pay close attention to our bodies in terms of their somatic knowledge—all the implicit and explicit knowledge they hold and the subtle and not so subtle changes in our energy levels—and manipulate that diet so it leads to a state of internal coherence. Put simply, we need to pay attention. We must pay attention to what may be healthy for us at very subtle levels and understand that negative thought patterns, words, and influences that on the surface may seem harmless actually perpetuate negative reactive patterns that permeate our bodies.

Also, conversely, we need to create those things in our lives that contribute to positive reactive patterns. We need to intentionally create internal coherence and do it often. The more we create states of internal coherence, the more those states become our way of being. Create abundance of positive influences in your life and do it often. The more often you experience positive reactive patterns, the more those neural networks and biochemical reaction patterns are strengthened. Pay attention to what is positive, and intentionally manipulate those outcomes with your words, choices, actions, and interpretations.

Using Your Body as a Gauge

Gravitating toward a state of internal coherence by taking notice of our physical reactions to specific stimuli requires us to pay close attention to the feeling response state of our bodies. By doing this, we need to be careful not to get caught up in the emotionally reactive response to which we may be accustomed. There needs to be a clear distinction between the concept of using our bodies as sensors for internal coherence and as an excuse for becoming emotionally reactive if we are out of coherence. The higher the state of internal coherence, the higher functioning we are. Emotionally reactive states cause internal chaos.

The goal of the energy diet is to work for a state of internal coherence by choosing or changing what we expose ourselves to and taking steps to maintain or improve that coherence as we make concrete changes in our lives. The higher the state of internal coherence, and the longer we maintain those states, the higher functioning and healthier we become, the more our whole lives become coherent. Furthermore, those choices should evolve as our coherence level improves.

We are all at different levels of development, in all different areas. Thus, it is appropriate to always pay attention to what is right for you in every circumstance. In paying attention and creating a positive energy diet, this chapter asks you to look at many different aspects and situations in your life. What may be an energy drain for you in one area may not affect another, and vice versa. What may be a negative somatic influence for one person may be fine for you. What may be a reactive situation for someone else may not necessarily affect you in the same way.

The important thing to remember is that somatic knowledge is knowledge that the body holds, usually because of a thought or feeling about something. It often can be subconscious. However, whether conscious or subconscious, the body is responding because of biochemical, neural, and electrical responses to that thing, thought, or situation. Additionally, remember that our brain synapse patterns fire in response to a thought or feeling, and this synapse firing may also be subtle. It is important to keep in mind the fundamental physiological changes that are occurring at each and every moment.

Increasing Cognitive Awareness of Harmful Patterns

If you are not used to or comfortable with tuning into the physical aspects of the energy diet, begin by processing what is likely happening from a cognitive standpoint. For example, by processing what negative language is likely to do to your brain neural networks, you may decide that language is something you need to consider in your energy diet. It may not come from a feeling state as much as from new understanding of the damaging process you are exposing yourself to with negative language, choices, and exposures.

In other words, you may decide that something is not healthy to expose yourself to because you now understand the damage you are doing to yourself with your current behaviors. I encourage you to apply this knowledge to all aspects of your daily life. How do you speak? What do you say to yourself all day long? Do you choose a negative interpretation of an event over a positive one because you have trouble allowing yourself to be happy? Do you allow yourself to get caught up in negative reactive patterns because you "deserve" to feel that way? Do you constantly expose yourself to situations that drain you of your life force? Conversely, do you routinely and intentionally incorporate events and circumstances into your life that increase your life force?

The answers to all of these questions powerfully affect your ability to cultivate transformation. If your life is full of chaos, or merely mundane and status quo events, that is what your brain is working hard to duplicate. Conversely, if your life is full of those things that substantially increase your life force, then that is what your brain is working hard to duplicate. The choice is yours. Pay attention.

Again, we all have different levels of development in all areas, and live from different levels of internal coherence. The challenge is to always pay attention to your own level of internal coherence, or energetic vibrations as Dyer would describe it, and work to raise those levels in yourself. Pay attention to the subtle and not so subtle shifts in your energy.

Process the information about brain conditioning and how this information is at play in every choice you make and every word you say on a daily basis. Assess the negative or positive shifts in your awareness or feeling states, even if you can't put words to them, and keep in mind the power this awareness can have on your own transformation. Listen for the "intuitive yes." Listen for the ineffable. Pay attention to your physical reaction and ask what will be added to or taken from your life force. Only you can interpret what these statements mean for you, and somewhere you have the answer.

A Story of Choice

Let me share a personal story that happened at the Esalen Institute, one of the most spiritual and healing places I have ever been. I was meditating as I was sitting on a cliff over the Pacific Ocean. I was dealing with some tough problems in my life and feeling that I was not living as positively as I would have liked to be living at the time. As I was meditating, I was hoping to get some answers to my questions, a positive direction in which to take some steps. As I came out of my meditation, I noticed a man standing nearby. I had not realized he was there. His name was Steve.

Steve asked me directly if I had had any important or profound insights reveal themselves as I was meditating. I was surprised by his presence, and I was surprised by his question because I had, in fact, had some very important insights. Most of all, I was surprised by the depth of the conversation that ensued. What I shared was this: I felt that if I could ask myself, every minute of every day, whether a choice was positive or negative, if I could take in to "feel" the answer from a deep and genuine place, and if I could pursue the only the positive, a substantial shift would take place. This idea was not new to me, but it was reaffirmed at a very deep level.

Steve shared a similar idea. He said he thinks that every decision or choice can be made out of love or out of fear. Those made out of love are the life-affirming choices, the ones that increase our life force. However, he added that it takes incredible strength and awareness to make only those based on love. I was reminded of the lyrics of a Bruce Springsteen song, "Cautious Man," that go something like this:

On his right hand Billy'd tattooed the word "love"
And on his left hand was the word "fear"
And in which hand he held his fate was never clear.

The concepts of love and fear can be overt and obvious, or subtle and implicit. In my opinion fear can be quite intimately connected with the ego, with feelings of "should," or who we think we need to be for external accolades because we are afraid to look inside ourselves. In other words, our choices are more motivated by fear of not being who we think we should be than by love and acceptance of who we are internally at our core.

The concept of an energy diet is to pay attention to both the big things and to the seemingly mundane things in our daily lives and to make a conscious choice to focus on the ones that for us create or enhance a higher internal experience. Some will base those choices on a feeling or somatic response, some will base those choices on a cognitive interpretation and synthesis of the information provided in this book, and some will know intuitively. You will know if you are willing and aware.

How Can You Tell? For 'Feelers' and 'Thinkers'

I am a "feeler." I can intuitively feel in my body when something is healthy for me or not. That "intuitive yes" or "intuitive no" is a whole body response for me. Some of that reaction is inherent; a lot of it is conditioned from knowledge I have gained through this process. The term that is often used for knowledge assessed by a feeling reaction is *somatic knowledge*. *Somatic* means relating to the body, and somatic knowledge has been the foundation of this book, as most of its focus has been on the physiological aspects of internal experience. Learn to tune into your body. Your body holds powerful knowledge of which you may or may not be conscious, as an extraordinary amount of physiological change occurs in response to what we are feeling and thinking.

If thinking in these terms is a new concept for you, doing so requires constant and vigilant awareness of how you are physically feeling and reacting due to certain circumstances. Additionally, it is important to synthesize the information you have gained throughout the process of this book in assessing that effect. You will be more aware of negative effects if you understand what is going on physiologically.

For instance, one of the things that I know is damaging for me is watching certain things on television. I know that watching some programs bothers me tremendously, and I definitely feel a reaction. My reaction goes beyond not liking those programs. Because I know that anything that intentionally manipulates my emotions in a negative way is creating the neural and biochemical patterns synonymous with that emotion, I am much more likely to be aware of my somatic or feeling reaction.

Because I understand the dynamics of what is going on in my brain, I am much more aware of my body. It is really a somatic and cognitive choice. More simply, because I understand the negative physical impact from poor choices, I am more likely to feel that impact. Additionally, I am quite aware from a reasoning level of the harm of a specific stimulus, and I am making a conscious choice to avoid that stimulus. In other words, I choose to avoid something because I have learned the negative impact it may hold for me.

If it still seems foreign to you to assess how you are physically feeling as a response to certain situations, think back to the emotion charting exercise in Chapter Five. In this activity you were asked to place what you felt were positive emotional responses above the line and negative emotional expressions below the line. When you are faced with a choice, think about this landscape. What feeling response are you likely to get from that choice? Is it above the line or below the line?

Remember these choices can be large or small in the scheme of what you would normally think of as an important choice in your life. However, the small choices, day after day, add up to large adaptations in your brain, body, and psyche. Picture those intravenous (IV) bags that hang next to the beds of hospital patients; the bags are full of medicines and fluids administered to patients via a needle in a vein. Now imagine yourself walking around all day long with two IV bags, one full of positive chemicals and the other full of negative chemicals. Every time you make a choice that is not life affirming to you, a drip comes from the negative IV bag. Every time you make a choice that is life affirming to you, a drop comes from the positive IV bag. Each drip creates a whole host of physiological reaction patterns experienced throughout your body and brain, complete with changing brain synapse patterns that influence future choices. Day after day, drip after drip, these little choices determine who we become.

Energy Awareness and Raising the Bar

Given all this information, how do we concretely create a positive energy diet? This section divides awareness of an energy diet into two parts. The first part emphasizes creating an awareness of all aspects of our lives that affect our somatic energy level either in a positive or negative direction. If a somatic reaction does not work for you, synthesize the information you have learned about possible physiological and psychological reaction patterns, and decide what should be healthy for you in those terms.

Part one of creating an energy diet asks you to pay vigilant attention to how you are responding to all aspects of your life, as demonstrated by your somatic or feeling response to all people, situations, things, places, relationships, and media. Pay attention, or, to return to a term examined previously, "become the observer." Remove yourself from emotionally reactive responses and make positive shifts in exposure whenever and wherever possible.

After paying close attention to your somatic or reasoning response in various areas of your life and after critically examining areas of your life that are likely influenced by negative neural or brain patterns, the next step is to shift to the positive. The second part of creating an energy diet asks you to find various ways to build into your life, on a constant and regular basis, those activities that substantially contribute to raising your positive physiologic or somatic energy level. Keep in mind every thought, feeling, action, or exposure you have creates a whole host of dynamic changes in your body, which ultimately determines your level of internal experience. Using the concept of an energy diet as a tool for transformation rests on the idea that the longer and more often you expose yourself to positive physiological, biochemical, and neural states, the more your body and brain adapts to those states and the more those states become who you are.

"Raising the bar"—that is, consistently and constantly exposing your body to what is positive for you in a psycho-physiological sense—is like somatic exercise for your life. As a result of physical exercise, your body changes by becoming more fit and making positive adaptations to live a healthier life. Most often, blood pressure decreases, body fat decreases, cholesterol decreases, cardiovascular and heart health improves. and the entire state of your physical body transforms.

In a positive energy diet, the biochemicals to which you are constantly exposed reflect a more positive state, your brain synapse patterns change to reflect more positive thought processes, and the plasticity of your brain begins to adapt and reflect a more positively functioning person. In short, you change.

Part two recognizes the fundamental importance of creating inspired activities as nourishment for your somatic health, a positive shift in brain patterns and whole body physiology, and asks how you can more effectively incorporate these activities routinely into your life. Dyer breaks the word *inspired* down to being "in spirit." What activities truly bring you to being in your own spirit? How can you consistently and routinely maximize your exposure to those activities?

Following are some specific areas and ideas that may help in concretely looking at specific choice patterns. This is by no means a complete list, nor is it meant to address every choice you make. It consists of two parts: (1) those things you may be exposing yourself to now and (2) ways or ideas to enhance, or "raise the bar," of your positive energy or vibrational levels for maximum exposure.

This approach is by no means meant to push or encourage change in someone who is not ready to make specific change. Nor is it meant to present these situations as if they are answers for everyone. These recommendations are merely an invitation to look deeply and honestly at your choices and to determine what is energetically healthy for you and what is not.

Every person is sensitive to different areas. Every person has a different level of energetic vibration, as Dyer would term it, and we each need to determine what is healthy for us. I personally believe there are some universal truths in the ways we treat others, but each person must honestly and genuinely discover these truths for himself or herself. These are some suggestions on where and how to begin looking and how to enhance exposure so that we may, on an energetic and somatic level, begin the transformative process.

Energy Diet Specifics

The purpose of taking concrete steps to create an energy diet is to pay careful attention to those things that may be affecting us somatically, or at the level of the body. It is important to pay attention to these things because everything we expose ourselves to, every person, choice, environment, thought, or reaction, carries a physiological reaction pattern that is either contributing to positive adaptations or negative adaptations that determine who we become, even though these reactions may be so subtle that we may not even be aware of them. This brings us back to the underlying theme of this book—that our internal experience basically creates who we are, that this can be documented and measured at the level of our physiology, and that intentionally cultivating positive or higher internal experience creates the foundation for change from the inside out.

These positive or negative reactive patterns can be measured in our biochemistry. They can be seen in our neural networks. You personally may not be adept at feeling these shifts as physiological reaction patterns, but they exist whether you are aware of them or not. The key is to be able to identify situations and circumstances that enhance or diminish those reaction patterns. Whether you do it by reasoning or by feeling is less important than truly learning to identify those situations in your life.

Keep in mind the most important aspect of identifying these circumstances is our internal experience of them, because our internal experience creates our physiological reality. When assessing the negative or positive impact of those situations in your life, think about your internal experience of them. Think about their physiological and neural impact, and imagine the process of what is occurring in your body and brain as a result of exposure to them.

One of the practices I find most helpful in this area is trying to always be aware of the emotional or psychological content of a situation to which my brain and biochemistry are exposed. In other words, if I am in a specific situation and I feel my emotions or thought processes are being affected or manipulated in a negative way, I am very aware in that moment of what this manipulation may be doing to my brain synapse patterns and biochemical reactions. I am also aware that the experience of these reactions contributes to long-term adaptations that may eventually affect my perceptions and behavior.

These situations can be as obvious as manipulative, toxic, or emotionally draining people or as subtle as exposure to specific forms of media, physical environments, or the act of taking responsibility for others' happiness. Whether obvious or subtle, the key to remember is that our personal exposure is measurable in our bodies, and by our choices we are creating our personal evolution.

People

Think of the people in your life. Do any of them, for whatever reason, seem to manipulate your emotions in a negative way? Are there those who want you to get caught up in their drama or listen to their never-ending tales of victimization? Pay attention to your response. There is a big difference between being empathetic and supportive and getting so caught up in others' experience that it becomes yours. Pay attention to your own reaction patterns. Are you beginning to react as if it is your experience?

My friend Laurie often says empathy is being able to put yourself in another's shoes—without making them your shoes. This is not to suggest that being supportive and empathetic is a bad thing. It is a recommendation to be aware of how you are affected by other people. On the most subtle level, some people you love and care about may have chosen to adopt, maintain, or wallow in a behavior pattern that you are beginning to assume as your own. Be aware of your own physiological adaptations and protect yourself against adopting the other person's negative neural patterns and biochemistry.

Our exposure to toxic people is an obvious example. We may feel physical or psychological responses just by being in their presence. The impact to our own physiology is very real; if we get caught up in anger, frustration, or disgust as a result of being in a relationship with these people, we suffer ill effects of that exposure, even more so if we have gotten caught up in our own reactive patterns. An all-consuming negative reaction to someone is much worse for our psychology and resultant adaptations than being able to remain neutral or disengage from that reactive state.

Many people will fall in between. We may find ourselves having a negative internal experience from being exposed to or in a relationship with someone. Since our repeated internal experiences become our reality, if the repeated experience is draining, toxic, or angry, our brains begin to strengthen those neural networks. Pay attention to your reactions to everyone with whom you come in contact. How are you responding? What are your subtle and not so subtle physical and psychological reactions? Can you reduce the contact with this person? If you cannot or choose not to, how can you disengage from adopting their negative reaction patterns?

Recent fascinating research regarding the action of mirror neurons underscores this concept. Mirror neurons are neurons in our own brains that appear to activate while observing an act performed by another exactly as if we were performing this act ourselves. Additionally, further research that this phenomenon exists was based on the mental understanding of an act beyond the visual observation.[4] In other words, if we allow ourselves to get too caught up in another's mental drama, anticipation of catastrophe, or constant chaos, the mirror neurons in our own brain may be reacting as if that drama is our own.

There is a vast and foundational difference between being genuinely compassionate, empathetic, and caring and assuming another's drama. We can be most supportive when we are able to remain internally coherent and centered and care from that state. Additionally, many times people we are in contact with want to stay immersed in their drama or their personal stories because there is some payoff for them in doing so. If we are experiencing true compassion, it should not drain our own personal energy. If it is draining, we need to rethink our boundaries. True compassion and loving kindness are some of the highest emotional states a person can cultivate and should produce positive reactive patterns within ourselves. Learn to cultivate these states without falling victim to the energy drain of another's behavior.

Media and Conversation

Everything we expose ourselves to creates and strengthens neural networks. What do you expose yourself to on a daily basis? Pay careful attention to the media in your life. What you watch on TV, movies, news, music, video games, the Internet—even listening to the town gossip—creates response patterns in your brain and body. If something is overtly or even subtly emotionally manipulative, your brain and body respond and adapt. Even something that on the surface may seem entertaining is creating important shifts in physiology.

We all have seen TV shows that capitalize on what seems to be the lowest common denominator of human behavior. Even if, on the surface, these shows seem entertaining, our brains and bodies are being exposed to those adaptations. The same is true of movies and some news shows, video games, and music. If we are having even a slightly lower emotional reaction, and that reaction could be delight at someone else's ignorance, we are being affected. The same is true of engaging in gossip or demeaning conversation in person or even in reading a magazine. When we choose to use hurtful, demeaning, or judgmental words, our own brains, bodies, and psyches are affected.

Environment

Our environment inspires subtle emotional reactions in us. These subtle reactions, of course, create neural and chemical reactions that may be beyond our awareness, except in a subtle shift in how we feel. Pay attention to your environment. This includes noise, physical space, simplicity, and distractions. In particular, be aware of your personal reactions and sensitivities to different aspects of your environment. Create nurturing, calming, and positive environments, and your coherence level will adapt accordingly. Question the places you routinely visit. Do they carry a positive response for you? Look at both the places you go every day and the places you choose to go for relaxation and vacation. Pay attention. The subtle reactions in your body certainly are.

Overloaded and Overwhelmed

When we are constantly functioning from overload and being overwhelmed, we are exposing ourselves to the negative physiological reactions and adaptations of constant chatter, catastrophizing and the moods that accompany those states. Just as importantly, we are not making room for positive states. Pay vigilant attention to where your emotional focus is. If you are constantly focused on feeling overwhelmed or overloaded, take big or small steps to refocus your emotional attention to a positive state as often as possible. Take short breaks and intentionally cultivate a shift by practicing the techniques presented in this book. This is a powerful way to change your perceptions of overload. Take breaks and experience something that for you can facilitate a shift. Look at the stars, go for a walk, talk to someone you love.

Sex

Human sexuality touches most of us very deeply. To examine the things in our lives that may contribute to a positive or negative energy diet without considering the tremendous impact of sex would be an incomplete conversation. Taking notice of how sexual relationships may affect our energy diet requires some background knowledge and a good degree of attention.

This section of creating your energy diet is separated into three components: (1) what may be negative for us, (2) attention to our "time budget," and (3) the intentional cultivation of the positive. Some may wonder why I have listed sex initially as a potential negative. I actually believe it can be an incredible positive, and in my opinion, sexual relationships can be one of the most spiritual ways one person can connect with another, but first some important considerations must be taken into account. The reason I initially list it as a potential negative has a lot to do with the way sex is quite often practiced. My feeling about the role sex plays in people's lives has much less to do with moral judgment than with the recognition of the chemistry of deep connection.

When a person is involved in sexual activity, especially when that activity culminates in orgasm, a large level of oxytocin is produced and released into the bloodstream. Sometimes referred to as the "bonding hormone," oxytocin is the hormone most responsible for creating the physical and psychological states associated with deep connection. When two people engage in sexual activity, according to Dr. Uvnas Moberg, oxytocin may serve to create a feeling of bonding or connection between them.[5] However, when people engage in sexual activity without connection to or regard for their partner, the encounter may be physically stimulating, but it is often followed by a sense of emptiness, loss, loneliness, or depression.

I believe this is the effect the oxytocin without the psychological connection it is designed to deepen. The body seeks to bond biochemically to a person or situation that does not warrant the closeness. I see this as a potentially tragic situation for many younger people, especially females who have adopted "hooking up," the new and accepted term for casual sex. Many of these people have not associated the feeling of emptiness afterward or the next day as a direct result of the chemistry of the sex act itself.

Another consideration is that sex is experienced in the brain mostly in the limbic system, close to and even partially overlapping the areas where we experience spirituality. I believe sex is designed to help us bond, connect, and feel biochemically and biologically varying levels of transcendence. To devalue sexual activity as anything less than transcendent may leave us with implicit or subtle levels of negative energy. Conversely, to celebrate the deepest levels of connection, bonding, and transcendence that sex can provide may be one of the strongest sources of positive energy available.

Uvnas Moberg contends that the intense oxytocin release during sex is designed to make us feel significant attachment to our partner. The message, again, is to pay attention. Pay attention to all aspects of how you feel before, during, and after sex. How do you feel the next day? Realize the profound biochemical changes taking place. Understand that biochemically we are designed to connect and bond with our sexual partners and create practices that honor and enhance that connection. Respect and revere the humanity of all involved and create practices that foster connection rather than detachment.

The next section deals with the concept of a time budget and how time exerts negative and positive influences in our lives. Then, we will examine a positive energy diet to intentionally cultivate higher internal experience and explore the importance of subjective interpretation.

Our Time Budget

There are many tools, techniques you can use and questions you can ask yourself to achieve the "energy diet" mode of thinking. One concept I find especially helpful is the idea of a time budget. The hours in a day are finite. How do you choose to spend those hours? Those minutes? Keeping in mind that time is finite and how you spend that time substantially determines whether your body, brain, and psyches are adapting positively or negatively helps to determine whether you are making wise "time budget purchases." If your goal is to experience significant transformation, then your days and hours need to be comprised of the things that will contribute to your positive development. Conversely, if your days and hours are comprised of mundane, subtle, and not-so-subtle negative influences, then you adapt to those experiences. When you keep in mind that adaptations are constantly taking place in response to what you expose yourself, your daily choices of exposure become very important considerations.

A central questions to ask yourself within the time-budget framework is: Are the activities (people, places, etc.) on which I'm choosing to spend my time life affirming? This question should elicit a feeling response. Only you can determine what is life affirming for you. As you consider that question, instead of analyzing or getting too caught up in the thought process of trying to answer, tune into your body. The feeling or emotional response most often initially comes from the subconscious part of your brain, so it is imperative that you learn to listen. Learning to listen in this context means listening to the subtle or implicit responses from your body. You know it because you feel it. Is it life affirming? Your body may know the answer.

The next step in the time-budget framework is reducing the time spent on those activities you don't deem to be life affirming. Part of recognizing what inspires you or what is life affirming for you is recognizing what does not inspire you or is not life affirming. Think of your life as a masterpiece in progress. Are you spending your valuable time contributing to that artwork? Remember the story of how Michelangelo created the statue of David in considering how to fashion the masterpiece of your life. Recognize what contributes to the true care and further positive development of yourself and chip away that which does not. Your time is precious, and your capabilities for transformation are, to a large extent, a sum total of the way you choose to spend your time. If your time is filled with those things that are less than optimal, that is what becomes the experience of your life. Conversely, if you spend your precious time on activities that are affirming for you, that becomes the experience of your life. Because repeated experience creates and strengthens neural networks in the brain, budgeting your time helps you create the richest experience you can in the time you are allotted, hour after hour, day after day.

Raising the Bar

Routinely and intentionally creating positive external circumstances that affect your internal experience provides the necessary conditions from which to grow. In other words, if you can routinely and intentionally create circumstances that truly and genuinely make you feel calm, coherent or internally happy, your repeated experience of these circumstances will change your body, brain, and psyche accordingly. These activities need to be what is most conducive to your own personal positive experience; however, the focus of the inner aspect of this experience is crucial.

Creating Connections

The powerful effects of oxytocin play a crucial role in the biochemistry of stress and the biochemistry of calm, connection, and trust. Earlier in this chapter, we discussed the release of this hormone during sexual activity, but oxytocin is also produced in any relationship based on emotional closeness and trust. We have substantial scientific evidence that oxytocin is produced when we create close and trusting bonds with others and that the production of this hormone lowers our stress levels and elevates our internal experience. There is incredible power in creating a supportive and connective community, whatever form that community may take. Connective and supportive communities actually have the power to change our biochemistry and resulting behaviors, neural adaptations, perceptions, and potential. There is power in intentional community. There is power in intentional connections.

Inspired Activities

We all have activities that nourish our soul or elevate our internal experience. These may be very different than the activities you simply enjoy. Allow yourself these activities. Allow yourself the deep experience that these activities may provide. Again, be willing to accept a higher internal experience. These activities are as individual as you are. They may involve a creative aspect or appreciating art. They may involve a stroll on the beach or a walk in the woods. You may find a higher internal experience by star gazing or swimming in a mountain lake.

Inspired activities may involve truly engaging yourself in something that resonates from the deepest part of who you are. If you are lucky enough, your work and your inspired activities are one and the same. Remember that Dyer breaks the word *inspired* into being "in spirit." What activities keep you in contact with your spirit? Are you truly willing to let these activities be part of your existence in such a way that you allow yourself to connect with that internal part of yourself? How can you routinely and consistently build these activities into your daily life?

Music, art, dance, communing with nature—these activities can stimulate an area in the limbic system that overlaps with the area of the brain we associate with spirituality. Inspired activities are truly a biological reality. Remember the premise of this book that we can achieve transformation by replacing negative activation of our limbic system with positive activation and in turn change our experience. Intentionally and routinely cultivating inspired activities creates change from the inside out.

Intentional Silence and Sacred Space

Creating sacred space can be a fundamentally important aspect of designing an energy diet. When we recognize that internal experience creates external reality, and elevating our level of internal experience substantially changes our physiology, behaviors, and perception, we can appreciate the power of sacred space. Having a designated space to which you can retreat, reenergize, and intentionally raise your level of internal and immediate experience can be invaluable in the transformative experience. This can be a designated space in your living environment, a place that you visit regularly for the purposes of a higher internal experience, or a sacred site as designated by a specific religious tradition. The key is to have this experience as a routine activity to truly create changes in your physiological response mechanism.

Intentional silence helps one cut through the chaos of daily life and intentionally get in touch with and create an elevated internal experience. Unfortunately, many people are so uncomfortable with who they are at the core that they do just the opposite. They fill their days, hours, and minutes with so much stimulation they lose touch with who they are at the core. Take a technology vacation. Remove yourself from the constant demands of cell phones, e-mail, text messages, Internet, and television. As my friend Violet says, get off the frantic treadmill and take time to look inside yourself. You may be amazed at what you see.

Honor Your Uniqueness

Each of us is unique. To be internally aligned is to recognize and celebrate our uniqueness. I was once in a conversation with a woman at Esalen. She was struggling with serious life decisions regarding her work and career. I mentioned I was writing this book, and we began to explore her struggles with her decisions. I could tell as she spoke that she was much more internally connected to one decision than the other; this was evident in her facial expressions, her body language, and her energy level as she talked through each scenario.

At the same time, she was trying to rationally talk herself into the other decision. I told her what a wise man once asked me: Is it possible to not do the thing that most resonates with you and still be happy at the deepest parts of who you are? I also asked her which choice she felt most passionately about and which most gave her that "intuitive yes." I shared my view that at our core we are all unique and we were given this uniqueness for a reason. If nobody else, at the deepest level, has the strengths and passions you do at your deepest level, are you not obligated to follow those passions? In creating your energy diet, follow your uniqueness, follow your passions, and create ways to weave them into your daily life and existence.

Be Open to Synchronicities and Coincidence

When you work on transformation from the inside out, you begin to cultivate the circumstances necessary to maintain that growth because your brain, beliefs, behaviors, and external actions begin to automatically respond to that transformation. Sometimes this cultivation appears in subtle ways. Pay attention. Know that your brain is functioning differently, and you need to take your transformation to a higher or more external level. Pay attention to synchronicities, pay attention to coincidences. In *The Spontaneous Fulfillment of Desire*, Deepak Chopra calls this "synchro-destiny."[6]

This is a popular and widely accepted concept today. Numerous books and programs explore the power of intention, or the process of attraction. Paying attention to synchronicities and coincidences is an important part of this process. Lately, it seems, when I put an intention in my consciousness, it manifests at the coffee shop I frequent! Part of creating these synchronicities and coincidences is holding the intention. Dyer encourages the practice of writing an intention or thought down on an index card, laminating the card, and either carrying it around with you where you are likely to always be aware of it (like in a pocket) or posting it where you will see it constantly. Constantly and positively focusing on the intention creates the physiological and neural synapse conditions necessary to manifest and receive that change.

Subjective Interpretation Can Make a World of Difference

One of my favorite quotes comes from Wayne Dyer: "When you change the way you look at things, the things you look at change."[7] Subjective interpretation, or the way we choose to see things, has a powerful effect on our emotional processing, our biochemical and brain reaction patterns, and our resultant ability to be genuinely happy. At first glance, subjective interpretation may not make sense, if we believe events are as they appear, and there is only one way to view them. I would argue, however, that most events carry some level of subjective interpretation, and most likely carry quite a bit.

Many times, in most situations, we have a choice of how to perceive or interpret that situation. Your interpretations and perceptions automatically change when you intentionally and routinely practice mental training to cultivate higher internal experience. New and more positive neural networks and brain synapse patterns have replaced the negative reactive patterns you previously functioned from, and your perceptions change as a result.

However, there is still a certain amount of subjectivity or choice in the way we view events. Intentionally choosing to focus on a positive interpretation activates and strengthens the associated networks, and we continue to transform our bodies and brains for higher potential, higher consciousness, and greater happiness. I am absolutely convinced that one of the most fundamental contributions to subjective interpretation is the level at which we are willing to allow ourselves to be happy. In other words, if we are truly willing to allow ourselves to be happy, we will automatically choose a more positive interpretation of events, or focus on the positive aspects of a situation rather than the negative aspects. This chosen focus activates and perpetuates associated physiological changes, and we begin to evolve in the direction of our interpretations.

Because talking about these terms in the abstract can be a bit confusing, I have included several stories to illustrate this point. These stories were purposely chosen to show how mundane situations can have a significant outcome because of the way we choose to interpret them. Also, because some of them are personal, they are not meant to sound arrogant in my own response patterns. One of the things I am eternally grateful for is how this transformative process has played out in my own life. I did not always choose positive interpretations and still have substantial room for growth, but I can honestly say that the level of happiness and genuine gratitude I experience on a daily basis has increased exponentially in my life since I began this process.

Some of these stories are everyday examples of the way we choose to view events and have the event itself totally transformed. Others involve significant outcomes or ongoing outcomes because of ingrained views of who we are. These go beyond the event itself because of major outcomes or in continuing negative and detrimental life behavior. However, they all began with a simple choice, in the moment, of how to view a specific event.

Once when my kids and I were on a road trip, everything possible seemed to be going wrong. One of the things we like to do most on long driving trips is listen to our favorite music. I had prepared the iPod we were using at the time for more than ten hours of great driving music. We left earlier than scheduled because I didn't want to be driving the dangerous two-lane highway in the dark and so we could make it to a place that would be perfect to spend the night. As we were heading into the desert, there weren't many choices.

Because we didn't begin the music right away, it wasn't until an hour into the trip that we discovered we didn't have the right adapter for the music, and seeing that we were heading into the desert, there were no places to stop to pick up the appropriate adapter. Trying to use this as an example for my kids, I kept pointing out all the positive things of the trip and actually encouraged them to look at all the things that were going wrong in a humorous light. After many hours of driving and experiencing many challenges along the way, we found ourselves in the pouring rain, in the middle of the desert, with no music to guide us. We also experienced a broken windshield wiper which I managed to fix with a spoon and a nail-clipper. Had my brain been flooded with cortisol, I would have never been able to dream that one up! When we arrived at our planned destination, we found a town with absolutely no vacancies in any hotel or motel within many miles.

At that point I really felt I needed music to keep me alert, because now it was dark, raining, and late at night on the very road I had tried to avoid in the first place. And, as my younger son tends to get very anxious when he is scared, I knew I needed to keep the mood positive. I dug through the car to find anything. All I could find was a very old, very corny CD with nothing but Christmas music on it (it was August). But we were having a great time. We were laughing at all the mishaps, singing at the top of our lungs to Christmas music in the middle of August, driving through the dark, in the pouring rain, through the desert to a town a few more hours away.

While this certainly wasn't a catastrophic event, all the little troublesome events along the way could have caused so much frustration that slowly but surely could have totally changed our perception of the event. The domino effect would have been in full force. If our perceptions had changed, each troublesome event would have increased our frustration exponentially (remember the mood congruency hypothesis), and soon we would have been having an absolutely miserable time, with all the physiological, biochemical, and neural effects to show for it.

This event happened when I was in the middle of writing this book so I was acutely aware of these dynamics. I was trying very hard to not allow the stressful shift in my body, knowing very well that if I did, it could be disastrous for both me and my kids, not to mention more dangerous if I got so stressed I couldn't think straight. The whole time driving I was completely engaged in intentionally letting myself feel the gratitude I have for my kids. I was happy, I was full of love, we were having a lot of fun, and I felt the difference in my total way of functioning. My kids did as well. It was an absolute intention to keep my focus on feeling this way. It would have been easy to let myself succumb to the anger and frustration of feeling victimized by the situation, but doing so would have only hurt myself and my children.

Another time when my kids and I were about to take a long driving trip, we were in the car, all packed, and the biggest spider that any of us had ever seen crawled up the back side of my seat. My youngest son is intensely afraid of spiders so we were delayed at least ten minutes while we were trying to find the spider in the car. We thought we had gotten it out of the car and drove on. When we stopped for gas later, the spider appeared again, and again we had another ten-minute delay.

At that point we had two options in regard to our subjective interpretation of the delay. We could have been frustrated and angry about the twenty-minute delay, which did ultimately affect our plans, or we could have been in charge of our own internal experience, and the circumstance, and chosen a different reaction. I tried to use the experience as a teaching lesson for the kids, so we made the effort to proceed with a positive attitude. By an odd coincidence, our run-ins with the spider prevented us from being involved in or at least witnessing a serious fatal accident on the same highway, in which a car was hit head on by a drunk driver about 20 minutes earlier. Even if we had not been involved personally in the accident, it would have been horrific for my kids to have come upon the scene any earlier as the bodies of the people who had been killed were still on the road and had just been covered up. We became very grateful for the delay that spider caused us.

I love talking about these issues with friends, acquaintances, students, and participants in my workshops. My friend Deborah shared the following story. She was about to take a long road trip with her two daughters. She had taken her car in to get a quick oil change, and in the process the mechanic noticed she desperately needed her tires replaced. She was amazed at how frustrated she was that her trip had to be delayed while her tires were repaired.

She was quite aware of the fact that having those tires replaced may have saved her and her children's lives, or at the very least a frustrating trip if she would have had a blown tire. She was also quite aware and questioning why her interpretation of the event was one of frustration and anger rather than gratitude for what had been discovered. Awareness of this process is the first step in being able to change those interpretations. Again, however, it is not just a cognitive activity; it most often requires a genuine feeling shift to create the associated adaptations in perception.

Many times our subjective interpretation or internal experience of an event will affect the outcome. One day on my way to work, I had a class starting at 9 a.m. and the lot where I always park my car was full, which had never happened before at that time in the morning. I could have easily become externally frustrated and began a downward stress spiral because I know the next closest lot was quite a distance away and I would be late to a class, which I never like to do. I happened to be handling things well that morning and decided there had to be a reason for the lack of parking space. I decided to see if a positive attitude, a cultivated positive internal experience, could change anything.

I found a parking place in a lot quite a distance away and walked to the building from a completely different direction than I would have otherwise. Outside the building, teaching golf in the rain, was my father, who also taught in the same department. Because I was operating from an internally coherent place, I was able to genuinely appreciate the circumstance. I wish I could accurately describe the warmth and love that spontaneously happened that moment. It was one of those moments that was seemingly random, but beyond words because of the loving connection that took place. Even though I was now even later to class, we had a quick, extremely heartfelt exchange in the rain that never would have been possible had I been in the negative internal space I could have been if I had let myself.

Walking down the hallway to my class, I had a wonderful feeling of love because of the exchange we had had and I felt that must have been the reason for the full lot. What I didn't realize at that moment was that would be the last time I saw him alive. He went home after class that day and had a massive heart attack and passed away. If I would have let myself fall into the frustration and anger that would have been so easy to succumb to when I couldn't park, I never would have been emotionally available for that type of exchange with my father. I would have prevented an extremely important event of my life.

Sometimes, subjective interpretation greatly influences the way we experience life as a whole. A student of mine, whom I have talked with extensively, struggles greatly with subjective interpretation. She only allows herself to be so happy and quite often subconsciously sabotages events by the way she interprets them, to keep herself in the role she perceives for herself. Quite often she makes comments like "that ruined the whole thing for me." She takes an event that may have been 80 percent or 90 percent positive, keeps the focus on the one negative aspect of that event, and completely invalidates everything that was good about it. In that way, she creates all the corresponding physiological adaptations of negative experience.

She quite often turns off emotionally to certain people or events, because in some way they touched on one of her trigger points, and then that situation or event falls into her paradigm of negative things "that always happen to me." What she doesn't realize is that by choosing to focus on the negative aspect, which is most likely coming from her own trigger points anyway, she is only perpetuating and strengthening the role she prescribes for herself.

If you find yourself turning off emotionally, abruptly from circumstance, honestly examine if there is another possible interpretation of events or a positive aspect of that event that you can carry instead of the negative. Honestly examine if you are willing, at a deep level, to allow yourself to be happy.

I need to be completely clear here that subjective interpretation does not mean suppression of appropriate emotional reaction. I once had someone very close to me make a poor choice that could have cost me my life. I understood the reasoning for that choice, but that reasoning certainly did not validate making the decision he did. But because I understood his reasoning, I never allowed myself to question or get angry. The problem with this suppression is that I carried it subconsciously for years. It was not until I let myself admit that it was an extremely poor choice, one that left me feeling very hurt, that I could begin to forgive.

Subjective interpretation, or how we choose to see things, can profoundly change what happens. When we interpret events, we create an internal experience of that event. When we have an internal experience of anything, that experience creates all the measurable changes in our bodies, brains, and psyches that have been the subject of most of this book. Subjective interpretation automatically improves when we do the physiological practices that were shared in Chapters Seven and Eight, but subjective positive experience can also be cultivated in its own right.

Subjective interpretation is about choosing to interpret events free from your trigger points. Subjective interpretation of events is about not falling victim to seeing the glass as half empty. It is about achieving higher potential and higher states of consciousness through a conscious choice of gratitude and other higher emotional states.

Conclusion

The topics covered in this chapter—our energy diet and subjective interpretation—complement and support the fundamentally important topics that have been covered in depth elsewhere. Personal habits such as exercise, diet, meditation, or other sustained mental practice, as well as the importance of semantics, have a great impact on our energy diet. Again, everything we do and say, every choice we make, and everything we expose ourselves to create implicit and subtle, or explicit and obvious, changes in our physiology. These changes influence our brain patterns, our perceptions, our behaviors, our future development, and our baseline level of happiness. Creating an energy diet is a personal practice to pay attention to how this concept is at play routinely and consistently in our daily lives.

Personal Energy Diet
EXERCISE AND REFLECTION #16

Reducing the Negative

Identify what, for you, are negative experiences. These experiences could be associated with people, places, environments, relationships, habits, exposure to certain types of media, or conversations. They will probably fall within all of these areas. Brainstorm, identify, and briefly explain as many situations as you can. The idea is to be very aware and identify all aspects of your routine experience that may contribute to subtle, or not so subtle, negative internal experience. After identifying as many areas that you can (and these areas will always change and evolve, so this list should be ongoing), brainstorm, reflect, and process on ways to reduce their presence in your routine experience.

_____

_____

_____

_____

_____

_____

_____

_____

_____

_____

_____

_____

Fostering the Positive and Creating a Time Budget

Brainstorm and reflect on ways that you can routinely incorporate intentional positive experience into your daily life. Focus on those activities that foster internal calm, coherence, and inner happiness, as these states are what promote internal growth. How do you create inspired activities? Sacred space? Intentional silence? Positive and nurturing connections? Focus on the inner aspect of these activities as specifically as possible, and identify ways to incorporate them into your life. Also reflect on your time budget. What are some ways you can spend more of your precious time on creating positive internal experience and reducing negative internal experience?

_____

_____

_____

_____

_____

_____

_____

_____

_____

_____

_____

_____

_____

Subjective Interpretation

Genuinely and honestly reflect on your tendencies in the area of subjective interpretation. Do you, at a deep level, genuinely allow yourself to be happy? Remember our interpretation of events is what fosters our repeated experience and resultant physiological and psychological adaptations. Many times, and most events, have some level of subjectivity, actually quite a lot if you look deeply and sincerely enough. I believe our subjective experience of personal events, or how we tend to look at things, is deeply rooted in how willing we are to actually allow ourselves sincere happiness.

Most of the time, we have a choice in how to interpret events. In all honesty, do you find you sabotage personal events or circumstances to "fit" your concept of how happy you think you should be or vice versa? Do you overreact to circumstances that don't warrant that response? How do your own personal reactive patterns play into this scenario? Do you find your personal reactive patterns routinely surface during important events? How can you disengage from your own reactive patterns if they are negative, and allow yourself a different experience? How can you foster positive personal reactive patterns to elevate subjective experience? In what areas do you routinely have positive subjective experience? In what areas can you improve? Reflect and process in a way that is meaningful for you, and keep in mind that the more honest you can be, the more transformation is possible.

_____

_____

_____

_____

_____

_____

_____

_____

_____

_____

REFERENCES

1. Orloff, J., *Positive Energy* (New York: New York Times Books, 2001).

2. Dyer, W., *The Power of Intention: Learning to Co-Create Your World Your Way* (Carlsbad, CA: Hay House, 2004).

3. Hawkins, D., *Power vs. Force: The Hidden Determinants of Human Behavior* (Sedona, AZ: Veritas, 1998).

4. Uvnas Moberg, K., *The Oxytocin Factor: Tapping the Hormone of Love, Calm, and Healing* (Cambridge, MA: Perseus, 2003).

5. Ibid.

6. Chopra, D., *The Spontaneous Fulfillment of Desire: Harnessing the Infinite Power of Coincidence* (New York: Harmony, 2003).

7. Hicks, E., and J. Hicks, *Ask and It Is Given: Learning to Manifest Your Desires* in Hicks and Hicks, p. xv (Carlsbad, CA: Hay House, 2004).

CHAPTER twelve

The Power of Semantics

The Power of Words

Words are powerful. Words come from thoughts and create more of the same thoughts. These thoughts result in corresponding neural synapses and strengthen the networks associated with those thoughts. Repeated thought patterns begin to ingrain the associated neural networks and become encoded as our way of thinking and functioning. In other words, the way we think and speak wires our brains to think more of the same and perceive and behave in accordance with those thoughts.

The focus of this chapter is on the power of words. The initial focus is on the words we say to ourselves, our constant personal chatter, catastrophizing and replaying our personal stories. The focus of the second part of this chapter is on the words we say, and how we say them, when we communicate with others. Semantics, or the words we use, are powerful determinants of who we are and the way we behave.

How do you speak to yourself? How do you speak to others? Which words you use, how you use them, what tone you employ, what your psyche tells you through your constant "inner chatter"—the totality of your communication—profoundly affects your thought processes and physiological response patterns. Again, every thought or feeling you have creates a cascade of biochemical, electrical, and neural reaction patterns that permeate your body. The words you use in communication with others and with yourself are powerful conductors of that physiologic cascade. In other words, the words you speak deeply determine who you are and who you are becoming.

The Words We Speak to Ourselves

Inner Chatter and Reactive Points

Pay attention to your constant "inner chatter." Is it predominantly negative? Is it predominantly positive? It is my experience that most of us carry predominantly negative "inner chatter" patterns. Does the inner chatter cause the thought or does the thought cause the inner chatter? The answer is both. Such is the circular nature of thoughts and brain response patterns, and unless we do something to interrupt those patterns we are caught up in an endless cycle of negative adaptations.

These adaptations in our brains only perpetuate the process, and it begins to become our conditioned automatic response. This is why, even when our attention is not intentionally focused on a specific thought, concept, or issue, we may notice the chatter happening automatically, like it is coming from some subconscious vault of response patterns. It is.

Remember the concept of emotional memory presented by Joseph LeDoux? Deep inside the brain, the amygdala serves as an emotional memory storehouse, tucking away enormous amounts of emotional memory response patterns.[1] It is important to remember that these patterns are subconscious reactive patterns, not the cognitive processing of the event, although that may happen simultaneously. Most often the emotional memory is experienced as a feeling, and that feeling may be processed as constant "inner chatter," and attached to whatever is present for us at the moment. In other words, something sets off a trigger in us, probably a situation or feeling that carries some characteristics of a stored reactive pattern, and immediately our chatter takes off.

Rhawn Joseph's research indicates that the emotional response patterns stored in the amygdala and limbic system are so enormous and numerous that the brain can only process "like" response patterns at a time.[2] This is consistent with LeDoux's mood concurrency hypothesis addressed earlier in this book. What all this means in connection to our own inner chatter is that, most often, that chatter is initiated by some conscious or subconscious trigger point, which unleashes a whole monologue of nonstop chatter that then reinforces the original feeling, whether or not that feeling was valid in the first place. The chatter becomes obsessive, and we are caught up in a perpetuating cycle of negative self-talk.

This concept may be easier to understand in the form of a story. When I am deeply honest with myself, I have to recognize that one of my deeper trigger points is the feeling of being rejected when I want personal attention. When I was growing up, my father was my hero, although he was not around or involved in my life in my younger years as much as I would have liked. I protected myself by constantly reminding myself that he really loved me, which was true, but he was just busy and had his own issues in being able to show love. However, I know somewhere deep in my brain is stored the hurt and emotional memory of missing him when he was not around.

This hurt seems to replay itself over and over again in my personal relationships. Something similar triggers this feeling, and immediately my free-floating emotionally reactive state needs to attach itself to that thing. I can feel my body responding with anxiety, fear, and anger. My whole body begins to tense, and I feel a sense of being overwhelmed.

When this emotional reaction comes up, I am absolutely convinced it is appropriate in the current circumstance.

Then comes the chatter. The chatter tells me all the things wrong with the current situation. The chatter tells me it is valid to feel the way I do. Chatter, chatter, and more chatter. The chatter creates more biochemical reactions to validate my point and creates more brain synapse patterns that reinforce my current thought processes and feeling reaction patterns. In all honesty, I can't tell if my response is appropriate for the current situation because my perception is clouded by the cascade of inner chatter and resultant physiological and psychological response patterns to that chatter. In short, my chatter has created my reality, and that reality may be distorted. The true reality is that if I didn't have my own stored reactive patterns, I probably would have perceived the event quite differently. Even if it still warranted action, action from a positive assertive place would be much more productive than action from a reactive state.

Although my story is used here as a demonstration of how this process works, the manifestation of this process occurs for each of us every moment of every day in all sorts of circumstances. Can you identify instances where it happens to you? You don't have to psychoanalyze the origination of the trigger point, or what creates the emotional memory in the first place, to stop this process. If you notice a strong emotional reaction, a reaction that seems to replay itself in similar circumstances, or a reaction that seems to set off a cascade of inner chatter or feeling of catastrophe, the emotionally reactive pattern is probably stored deep in your brain, and the magnitude may or may not be appropriate for the circumstance. In either case you need to "own" it and not let the chatter take you on a physiological downward spiral.

It is important to note that you still may have a negative assessment of the situation or feel your feelings are legitimate. However, if you come from a less emotionally reactive place, one free of negative inner chatter or feeling of catastrophe, you will have a much clearer perception or assessment of the current situation and make a more sound decision about what is right for you and your needs. In my own story, turning off the chatter and feeling of catastrophe, disengaging from the emotionally reactive place, and recognizing my own propensity to exaggerate those feelings allows me to make a more emotionally coherent decision about what level of engagement is best for me.

Psychoanalyzing—that is, trying to identify the trigger's origination point—is not necessary and in many cases may not be beneficial if that process keeps you stuck in victim patterns. Figuring out the origination point may be helpful under certain circumstances; however, not letting yourself get caught up in and be defined by that reaction pattern is the most important step in the transformation process. In other words, if you take the time to figure out what causes specific triggers in you but choose to remain stuck in those patterns of reaction because you feel validated if you do, knowing the source doesn't do any good.

A good example of this is the feeling of "that is what so-and-so used to do" or "this is what always happens to me," and yet allowing yourself the same response and maybe even validating it because of your past experience. Knowing the source is most beneficial when you use that knowledge to grow beyond those reactive patterns. Paying attention to physiological and psychological reaction patterns to any and all circumstances is the key. Listen to your inner chatter. Are you becoming upset, tense, anxious, or angry? Does the feeling and sound of the chatter feel familiar? Are there other situations that set off this same feeling or reaction in you? Does the current thought or circumstance that is triggering the chatter bring up all sorts of negative memories or feelings? Can you disengage from the chatter?

As Joe Dispenza suggests, become the observer.[3] Remove yourself from the emotionally reactive state, recognize that the emotional reactive pattern is something physiologically stored and released deep in your brain, and turn off the chatter by refocusing your emotional attention. Understand that the chatter re-creates and reinforces our reaction patterns and, in essence, keeps us addicted to those patterns.

Notice your chatter. What do you say to yourself all day long? How do you talk to yourself? Are you constantly putting yourself down or questioning your worth in certain situations? Are you constantly looking for external validation and falling into negative chatter against yourself or another if that validation doesn't come? Do you replay situations over and over in your head of what you could have said in a certain situation? Do you chatter about all the things that could go wrong? Do you automatically imagine catastrophe?

Catastrophizing

Catastrophizing, that is, always imagining the worst that could happen in a situation—is an especially destructive type of internal chatter. When people anticipate catastrophe, they play scenarios in their heads of all the things that could go wrong, all the things that might go wrong, or all the ill intentions that someone may have against them. In their defense, people who embrace catastrophe may claim the cliché that they are "preparing for the worst, but hoping for the best." However, when looked at honestly, that preparation involves imagining little catastrophes that may or may not happen.

The problem with this outlook is that the brain and body perceive imagined situations and circumstances as if they were real. The more vividly we imagine a negative scenario, the more we biochemically and neurally respond as if that scenario had happened. Most of the time, the anticipated catastrophes never occur, but yet the wear and tear on our bodies and brains is very real. Because of the adaptations of the negative thought process, we have actually made our bodies and brains more capable of creating the same catastrophe or scenario we fear.

Lack of trust is one form of catastrophizing. Keeping our focus on all the ways we fear someone will violate our trust only makes us more biochemically and neurally capable of mistrust. Again, every feeling and thought we have and every choice we make create a cascade of biochemical reactions throughout our body. Although it seems easier to comprehend the negative biochemical reaction patterns, there are also biochemical reaction patterns taking place with every positive feeling and thought we have and every positive choice we make. The same is true for trust, and there is compelling research to support this concept.

Zak, Kurzban, and Matzner researched the "bonding" hormone oxytocin in relation to trust. In a blind experiment, they found that people who made the choice to trust and those of who received that trust produced higher levels of oxytocin. The research participants made a voluntary choice to trust, not knowing anything at all about what was being measured in the experiment, and that choice created a very measurable and very positive biochemical shift in their bodies and the bodies of those who were trusted.[4] The message is that our choices create measurable biochemical realities in our bodies that then perpetuate what we perceive those realities to be.

In the chatter of mistrust and catastrophe, we play and replay the imagined scenarios complete with our created physiological reaction patterns that only make those scenarios more likely to occur. Even if, in the end, those scenarios don't occur, the wear and tear on our bodies and in our brains is very real. This wear and tear keeps us in status quo and severely limits the transformative process.

Replaying Our Stories

When something negative happens, do you constantly replay the story, situation, or circumstance over and over again in your head? How often do you retell the story to willing listeners so they can commiserate or share the dramatic effect? Do you somehow become the product of your stories? Retelling, recreating, or replaying a story to deal with it and release it from your consciousness is very different than retelling, recreating, or replaying a story for the dramatic effect. In all honesty, does part of you thrive on the drama or feel comfortable in the stress it produces?

Replaying our stories perpetuates and re-creates the neural patterns and biochemical patterns of the experience almost as if the experience were happening again. Also, recall what impact any repeated experience have on our bodies, brains, and psyches. Constantly replaying any event, or any negative interpretation of an event, only furthers to "hardwire" the propensity for like events in our reactive patterns and to wreak havoc on our psychophysiology. I've heard it said, "You are not your stories." This maxim holds great truth in the physiology of the transformative process.

Retelling our stories for the purposes of wallowing or perpetuating the victim attitude also creates neural and biochemical reaction patterns similar to anticipating catastrophe or negative chatter. Actually, replaying may be more harmful because a recalled experience generally brings up more vivid emotional responses. I find easiest to demonstrate the negative impact of replaying or retelling for sympathy in the form of a personal story.

Several years ago, before I learned to tremendous impact our thoughts and feelings have on our physiology and psyches, I was caught up in the following pattern: At my previous teaching position, I had a very toxic department chair. He was toxic to most everybody in the department, and some people even left their jobs to get out of that environment. He was famous for creating altercations with almost everyone with whom he came in contact, and from what I know now, even one altercation produces a substantial cortisol rush. As you may recall from previous discussions, cortisol is a damaging stress hormone and has a twelve-hour half-life. In other words, after twelve hours, it only takes one-half of the original dose to elevate the body back to the level caused by the previous stressful event.

There were some challenging issues concerning our department at the time, issues that were very near and dear to my heart and about which I had passionate feelings. As our department chair was prone to say things without thinking, one run-in with him would leave me feeling that my job and the program I had helped to create were both in jeopardy of being eliminated. Needless to say, because this was such an emotional issue for me, a five-minute conversation with him in the morning would flood my body with cortisol and other stress hormones and send my brain reeling with "what ifs," anticipation of catastrophe and negative chatter, complete with all the associated brain synapse patterns.

If I could have refocused my emotional attention right then and there, I could have saved myself from several hours of substantial emotional reactive physiological patterns and all the negative adaptations that accompany them. What I did instead was anticipate catastrophe. What I did instead was replay the altercation over and over in my head all day long, including all the horrible resulting scenarios I could imagine. What I did instead was send cortisol shots throughout my body all day long like an IV drip primed by my negative thought processes. What I did instead was activate negative brain synapse patterns repeatedly all day long with the result of strengthening those same reactive patterns.

In the evening, nearly ten hours later and after ten hours of low-grade "cortisol baths" and negative brain synapse patterns, I would have my chance to replay the drama. Of course, I wanted my husband at the time to feel sorry for me and relate to the negative emotional reaction and fear I had regarding the situation, so I would retell my story. However, I wasn't retelling the story to process it and figure out solutions, or process it and let it go. I was retelling my story to replay the drama. I was retelling the story to bask in the fear and negative possibilities and to get sympathy from my husband, so he could relate to how I felt victimized.

The problem with this retelling is that the more vividly you relive an experience, the more your body, brain, and biochemistry react as they did during the original event. In many cases, your brain can't tell the difference between the real and imagined event. Ten hours after the original event, I was producing at least enough cortisol by retelling my story to go back to the level of the original event, which would give me another twelve hours of cortisol. In essence, I had produced enough cortisol through my reliving, retelling, and anticipation of catastrophe to last me for twenty-four hours, just enough time to have another altercation the next morning.

All this reliving, retelling, and anticipation of catastrophe did nothing to help me deal with the problem constructively, but the wear and tear on my body and psyche were tremendous. Most of the horribly imagined scenarios never materialized, but I felt more beat up and stressed out that I had ever in my life to that point. Retelling for the purposes of letting go is far different than retelling to re-create. Armed with this information, now I have adopted the practice of saying, if I have determined it is important enough to share, "I want to 'vent' and then let it go."

Had I known then what I know now, it could have been very different. Had I known then what I know now, I could have saved myself many hours of the severely damaging effects of cortisol, and I could have saved myself many hours of repeated experience in negative neural and brain response patterns. Had I known then what I know now, I could have taken notice and refocused.

Notice and Refocus Your Inner Chatter

As has been stated many times, in many ways, all the knowledge put forth in this book will not support the transformative process if it is not put into action. Stress is an experience. Anxiety is an experience. Staying stuck in our current patterns of self-limitation, negative inner chatter, mistrust, and anticipation of catastrophe are all experiences. Beginning the transformative process of changing our bodies and brains by turning inward and paying attention to semantics must also be an experience.

How do you stop the negative inner chatter? How do you stop the catastrophizing, or automatically replaying all your negative stories? Take notice and refocus. Make it a point to stop several times a day and notice your thought patterns. Notice your energy or anxiety levels in regard to your thought patterns. Are your thoughts full of negative inner chatter? Are you constantly putting yourself down or doubting your worth? Are you constantly angry because you think someone else is not recognizing your worth? Are your thoughts routinely focused on the mistrust of others and how you perceive they are intentionally, or unintentionally, out to "get" you?

Set up a concrete plan and schedule to remind yourself to check your thought process. It could be every time you perform a certain task. If you drive a lot, it could be every time you come to a red light or stop sign. You could pick time reminders like very fifteen minutes on the hour, every time you eat, or every time you sit at a computer.

The way you make a schedule is not important. The idea is that you plan ahead for ways to remind yourself and build into your schedule reminders to pay attention to your thought process. Put a note on your mirror at home. Put a small note on your rearview mirror. Put a note on your desk or your computer. Write a note on a small index card and carry it in your pocket.

The message could be a simple question: "Where are your thoughts?" The key is to devise a concrete plan that works for you and your lifestyle, to have constant reminders to check your thought process. Once you become accustomed to this activity, it becomes a natural process. In other words, it becomes a natural process to be aware of where your thoughts are. When they are consumed with negative inner chatter, mistrust, anticipation of catastrophe, or replaying negative stories, your body serves as an alarm system to alert you and remind you to refocus your emotional attention. Take notice. Refocus.

The second step in taking notice is honestly asking yourself if the thought process is serving you. The key in this second step is absolute genuine honesty with yourself. Keep in mind the biochemical and brain reaction patterns your body is undergoing with every thought or feeling you have. If you are stuck in negative inner chatter, mistrust, catastrophizing or replaying negative stories, the chance for transformation is small.

There is a chance the negative chatter is a message that you have a specific issue you need to confront. Taking notice and dealing with the issue is a concrete step to using the negative inner chatter as a tool for growth. Only you, from a deeply sincere and honest state, can decide if the negative inner chatter is a push for growth or a trigger from your emotionally reactive center in your brain, your "baggage" center.

Regardless, staying stuck in the emotionally reactive place of negative inner chatter, mistrust, anticipating catastrophe, and replaying negative stories limits our transformative process. After taking notice, ask if the chatter is serving you. If it is not, refocus your attention to something positive. Intentionally "feel" one of the emotions you have listed on the top half of your emotional chart. If it helps to hold an image of something that helps you create that feeling state, do so. Remember it is the feeling not the image that is important, but the image or images you hold are useful tools in creating that feeling.

If you feel the negative inner chatter is a message of something you need to deal with, then disengage from the emotionally reactive state, stop the chatter, and take concrete steps to deal with that situation or issue. Taking concrete steps to resolve an issue contributes to the transformative process. Staying stuck in negative inner chatter does not.

In summary, all our negative inner chatter, catastrophizing, mistrust, and replaying of negative stories impair our transformative process. All of our thoughts, feelings, and actions create a cascade of biochemical and brain reaction patterns that negatively affect our brains and bodies and become who we are. Steps for transformation through the concept of self-talk or inner chatter can be easily remembered in the saying "take notice/refocus."

In the notice process, it is helpful to make some sort of a schedule or reminder system to help you constantly asses what is going on with your thought processes. The following journal activity will help you create a specific plan that is appropriate for you.

The take-notice process also involves genuinely and sincerely examining the content of the chatter. Is it coming from the emotionally reactive place in your brain? Is it part of your stored negative emotional memory system? Do you need to "own" it? Is it part of your own emotional baggage? It takes honesty, humility, love, and trust for yourself to recognize when it is and take responsibility for your own reaction patterns.

The refocus process involves making an intentional shift in your emotional attention. Make a specific intention to disengage from your stored negative reactive patterns and practice the refocusing tools presented in Chapters Seven and Eight. Pick what for you is on the top half of the emotional ladder and honestly feel that emotion. Use an image to help you create that feeling if it is appropriate. Let the negative chatter go, refocus your emotional attention, and start creating positive brain reaction patterns to replace the negative that are causing the inner chatter.

If, after careful assessment, you believe the negative inner chatter is an impetus for change, then the refocus process involves taking concrete steps to solve that issue from a clear-headed and emotionally coherent place. Refocusing your emotional attention by intentionally making a shift to a positive feeling state will help you think more clearly to determine the source of the inner chatter. Refocusing your emotional attention to higher states will help you decide what positive steps you need to take if that chatter is a push for change.

Take Notice

1. Set up a plan to constantly be aware of your thought process. Are you full of negative inner chatter, anticipation of catastrophe, or replaying of negative stories?

2. Is that thought process serving you or just serving to create more negative response patterns? Is it a message for change?

Refocus

1. Practice the exercises to refocus your emotional attention.

2. Make a plan, if necessary, to solve the issue creating the emotional reactive chatter.

Turn off the negative chatter and discover the possibilities present in the calm internal experience of silence. Instead of catastrophizing, picture possibilities. Instead of replaying negative stories, replay positive stories. Allow yourself to begin to trust. Your biochemistry and brain will thank you by adapting and beginning to transform to higher levels of internal experience.

Notice and Refocus Your Inner Chatter
EXERCISE AND REFLECTION #17

What is your typical negative chatter? In what areas of your life do you tend to automatically anticipate catastrophe? What stories do you retell, and under what circumstances are you likely to retell them? How can you remind yourself to check your inner chatter? What "sets you off" in an emotional reactive pattern, and how can you learn to disengage from the chatter that follows? The more specific you can be about catching these processes, the more likely you will be to overcome them and begin to retrain your self-talk reactive patterns. Remember, these patterns powerfully influence the neural firing in your brain and biochemistry. Reflect and process in a way that is meaningful to you.

_____

_____

_____

_____

_____

_____

_____

_____

_____

_____

_____

_____

The Words We Speak to Others

We often sabotage relationships in the ways we speak to each other. Words carry powerful brain reaction patterns associated with them, and every time we use hurtful or harmful language, those brain reaction patterns are strengthened in both the speaker and the listener. The power of semantics resides in cultivating positive language with others.

Words themselves can be violent because of their influence on our reactive patterns and emotional responses. If we remain acutely aware of this fact, we are less likely to revert to these patterns in an emotional situation. When we use blaming or accusing words, words that have an explicit or implicit moralistic judgment, or words that compare or deny our own responsibility, we are not using words that are conducive to higher internal experiences.

Additionally, what we know about biochemistry, the positive effects of oxytocin, and the damaging effects of cortisol underscores this point. Oxytocin is the bonding and connection hormone. Cortisol is the stress and anxiety hormone. What type of language we use powerfully affects our connections and relationships. It powerfully affects our capabilities of producing oxytocin, and thus strengthening immediate and long-term connections, or producing cortisol and intensifying feelings of alienation and disconnection.

In *Nonviolent Communication: A Language of Life,* Marshall Rosenberg identifies specific types of communication that block compassion. He includes in this "life-alienating communication" moralistic judgments, comparisons, denial of responsibility, demands, and statements that someone "deserves" a negative outcome or punishment. He calls this "the language of wrongness" and asserts that this type of language encourages people to look outside of themselves for roots and causes rather than be in contact with their own feelings and needs.[5]

For our purposes of transformation, it is especially important to underscore Rosenberg's association with people looking outside of themselves with negative or accusing language, as opposed to looking inside themselves to identify their own feelings and needs. Additionally, it is important in our considerations to emphasize the physiological aspect of language. A word flows from a thought and then creates more thoughts. If our words are condemning, judgmental, or moralistic, words coming from and creating lower emotional reactive patterns, then that is what is perpetuated as our way of being. If words are based on higher emotional reactions, then that is what is encouraged and perpetuated as our way of being, even down to the level of our cells. It is fundamentally important that we be mindful of the mind, body, and spirit connection in our choice of words. we can't create higher internal experience, and repeat those experiences, when our words are coming from lower emotional reactive patterns.

How can these concepts be applied concretely? Be acutely aware of your language. Avoid condemning phrases like "you do this, " "you do that," "you're too this," or "you're too that." Chances are, that if the statement starts with "you" or "you're," it is a condemning or judgmental statement. Condemnation and judgments come from lower emotional states and have no place in the process of transformation or positive semantics. Remember the absolute harm we are doing to ourselves, our brains, our bodies, our psyches, and our spirits when we allow ourselves to speak from harmful and lower emotional states.

Pay careful attention to your words. Usually words or statements that begin with "I feel" or "I need" are more genuinely based on positive internal experience, an experience that is based on expressing needs and desires without blaming or condemning in the process.[6] Pause, reflect, choose your words carefully, not from a manipulative way, but from a state of higher emotion and higher consciousness. Examine the typical words and phrases that for you come from lower emotional states and make plans ahead of time to avoid those words.

Use the notice, refocus, and choose techniques from HEART in communication with others. If you are in a discussion where you can feel emotional reactive patterns beginning to surface, remember the discussion of emotional trigger points. Notice your reactive patterns and disengage from them. Refocus your attention and choose a higher reaction pattern. Pause and reflect on what your sincere feelings and needs are in the situation, instead of using condemning, judgmental, or accusatory words.

This is a complete paradigm shift from the way we usually communicate, and it takes sincere willingness to disengage from the reactive semantics to which we are conditioned. Remember the acronym for the higher emotion and refocus techniques is HEART. Go to HEART and choose a different response. Sincerely focus on and express what your underlying feelings and needs are. Your brain, your body, and your spirit will reap the benefits. Transformation and higher states of consciousness are greatly enhanced by the power of positive and caring semantics.

Positive Communication with Others
EXERCISE AND REFLECTION #18

What are some likely circumstances in your own life that could benefit from positive semantics in relation to another? Be acutely aware of your language. How can you avoid condemning phrases like "you do this," "you do that," "you're too this," and "you're too that"? Identifying these circumstances ahead of time will help you transform the experience as it occurs. Do you routinely fall victim to negative communication patterns? What may be your underlying feelings and needs in these situations? How can you honestly express those instead of falling victim to destructive patterns? Keep in mind the physiological and psychological implications of routinely engaging in positive rather than negative communication.

_____

_____

_____

_____

_____

_____

_____

_____

_____

_____

_____

_____

REFERENCES

1. LeDoux, J., *The Emotional Brain: The Mysterious Underpinnings of Emotional Life* (London: Orion Books, 1998).

2. Joseph, R., *The Transmitter to God: The Limbic System, The Soul and Spirituality* (San Jose, CA: University Press, 2001).

3. Arntz, W., B. Chasse, and M. Vicente, *What the Bleep Do We Know!?* (Deerfield Beach, FL: Health Communications, 2003).

4. Zak, P. J., R. Kurzban, and W. T. Matzner, "Oxytocin Is Associated with Human Trustworthiness," *Hormones and Behavior,* 48 (2005): 522–527.

5. Rosenberg, M., *Nonviolent Communication: A Language of Life* (Encinitas, CA: PuddleDancer Press, 2005).

6. Ibid.

CHAPTER thirteen

Putting It Together

The major premise of this book is that deep and sincere transformation must come from within. Transformation must come from the deepest parts of ourselves, our internal experience, and as a result that repeated internal experience creates foundational changes in our bodies, our brains, our consciousness, and our lives. Like a pebble on a still pond, the initial impact reverberates out, and soon the whole pond is full of ripples from the original union of the pebble and the pond.

We began our journey to lasting and fundamental change by examining the process and chaos of stress, anxiety, and negative emotional reactions and how those reactions contribute to negative internal experience. Understanding the harmful impact of negative reactive states sets the stage to explore the tremendous possibilities of positive emotion and how the routine experience of these states actually changes the structure and functioning of the neural networks in our brains and the chemical composition of our bodies. Repeated experience, whether positive or negative, creates and strengthens neural networks in our brains. As Joseph LeDoux says, "We are our synapses."

The core of this book—the center of our metaphorical labyrinth—is the techniques designed for repeated experience of higher emotion. Our bodies adapt to what we give it, even down to the level of our cells. The Higher Emotion and Refocusing Techniques are designed to encourage us, in a routine and consistent way, to replace negative reactive states with those of higher emotion, those often associated with states of higher consciousness. By routinely experiencing these states, in the moment of stress as well as in sustained practice, we create measurable and fundamental changes in the way our bodies and psyches operate.

I have often heard and read that because of the rate at which our cells die and regenerate, we are literally a different person every seven years. Whether this is true or not, the impact of creating fundamental changes in the way our bodies process either lower or higher emotional states cannot be understated. Routine intentional and cultivated experience of higher emotional states, those of a higher internal experience and often associated with higher states of consciousness, are essential to transformation. When we notice, refocus, and choose a higher emotional response, a response based on love, care, compassion, kindness, and regard for the humanity of others, we fundamentally change, even down to the level of our cells. In my opinion, there is nothing more potentially transformative of our bodies, our brains, our psyches, and our lives than routinely making a conscious choice to get in touch with and operate from higher emotional states.

As with the ripples on a pond, the impact of these fundamental changes begins to reverberate out to our external lives. However, as in any area of behavior change, we must move from contemplation to action. These concepts will not contribute to our transformation if we merely know about them without truly engaging in their practice. We need to go to the source, we need to go to the root for growth or transformation to be successful.

The metaphor I think is most appropriate here is one of a tree. The root and the trunk are representative of our internal experience. The various branches are the external circumstances in which we live our lives. Without a healthy root system and trunk, the various branches will not survive for long, even if they appear to be experiencing healthy growth at any specific moment in time. The root and the trunk are the deepest parts of ourselves. If we begin by focusing on the health and nourishment of the base, or of our internal experience, the branches will blossom accordingly.

The routine and intentional practices of the techniques presented in this book, or other similar mental training techniques that focus on the intentional cultivation of higher emotional states, are what create and nourish the roots and trunk. From a fundamental change of who we are at the deepest levels of internal experience, the branches of healthy and productive external experience, full of higher potential, begin to grow.

After our examination of these techniques and their practical application, we considered the tough questions of willingness. Willingness is what attaches the roots and the trunk of internal experience to the branches of external experience. We must examine whether we are truly willing to allow change. The word *allow* is intentionally chosen because after fundamental internal change, external change is automatic, if we allow or permit it to take place. Are you willing to cultivate the external circumstances of your life to be conducive to, encourage, and sustain positive internal experience? Without willingness and allowance, transformation is just a concept.

"Tilling the soil" is about the cultivation of basic external practices that allow internal experience to flourish. It is about taking care of ourselves at some basic levels to help us be more in touch with positive inner feelings. If we physically feel better, we are better prepared for external growth, and we are better prepared to take care of the external demands of our lives.

Usually, when you board an airplane, the flight attendant gives you instructions about oxygen masks and how they work. He or she tells you that if you are traveling with a small child or someone else who might need assistance, you must secure your own mask first before you attempt to help another. You are instructed to secure your own mask first so you are better able to help another; for if we are suffocating ourselves, we can't help anyone else. Tilling the soil is about knowing what we need to do and taking concrete action to best take care of ourselves at the most basic of levels, so we can then function optimally.

Tilling the soil is about preparation. When we are physically and psychologically ready, change will come. It's like the old adage "the teacher will appear when the student is ready." I deeply believe in the contemplative experience of physical preparation. In other words, if we do what we need to do to prepare ourselves physically, not to reach some external physical ideal but because when we feel better we are less chaotic internally, we are much better prepared for change. Additionally, focusing on simplicity and meditation, or like practices, we are much less distracted by a chaotic life and environment and more able to focus on a richer internal experience.

What does tilling the soil mean for you personally? We all have personal practices we must foster to keep us much more grounded, centered, and feeling more internally coherent. When a gardener tills the soil, he or she pays loving attention to what may look like nothing more than dirt. But the gardener knows that with enough love, attention, and nourishment, that dirt is full of potential. With enough love and attention, that soil can become a blossoming garden. Additionally, the garden is always growing, changing, and evolving. Constant and ongoing attention to the quality of the soil is a must if the garden is to continue to flourish.

Beyond our own personal preparation, we began to look at some of the external circumstances in our lives that may profoundly and deeply influence our internal experience without us realizing it. Our "energy diet" encompasses all our daily experiences, including various situations in our lives that may be detracting from positive internal development. We examined the application and synthesis of the knowledge presented in this book and how we might use that knowledge to cultivate positive external experience that is more conducive to higher internal experience. In other words, we took what we learned about the very real biological implications of our life choices and examined how we can concretely create situations in our own lives to enhance our transformation.

We examined how for some that knowledge may be manifest more somatically, or felt in the body, and how others may gain more by reasoning how the information presented would play out in various circumstances in their day-to-day life. We considered the idea that the internal quality of our everyday experience has a cumulative effect and how this cumulative effect profoundly changes us at the deepest of levels of our brains, cells, and psyches.

We considered various situations in our lives that may add to or subtract from our repeated level of internal experience and reflected on ways to intentionally cultivate more routinely positive and higher internal experience. Various considerations were on the influence of people, places, and things in our lives that may have a positive or negative influence. We examined the importance of creating connections, the influence of environment, the detrimental aspects of being overloaded and overwhelmed, the importance of all relationships, and the concept of a positive and purposeful "time budget."

Intentionally cultivating positive experience included, among other things, honoring your uniqueness, creating inspired activities, seeking intentional silence and sacred space, and being open to synchronicities, coincidences, and positive connections. The underlying theme of creating these intentional activities is creating space and time in your life to gain access to your internal self and create positive experience from which to grow. Also of extreme importance to the cultivation of positive internal experience is the importance of subjective experience, or how we choose to see things or events, and the power of semantics.

The theme of this book is that growth must take place from the inside out, and now, at its culmination, we must look at the process of growth itself. This book is full of concepts; you must decide what works for you and what doesn't. I encourage you to reflect deeply. On the surface something may seem not to resonate, but at further glance it may fit perfectly now or at some future time or level of transformation. Allow yourself to be open. Be willing to see things differently. Remember, it's the internal experience that is paramount.

Also, take a very close look at those things you tend to resist. It has been my experience, throughout many years of teaching and presenting the concepts in this book, that those most resistant are quite often those who are just about to make foundational change. I have seen resistance give way to transformation many, many times.

At the very least, I hope you deeply entertain the information about the physiological adaptations your brain, body, psyche, and consciousness go through as a result of what you routinely give them. You have a choice not to react from lower emotional reactive states. You have a choice to notice, refocus, and choose reactions based on higher emotional states. Routinely experiencing higher emotional states leads to higher potential, higher internal experience, a higher baseline level of happiness, and higher consciousness.

Out of the Labyrinth

Now as we come out of the labyrinth that was the journey of this book, we look at the process of growth. The transformative process presented in this book can be as minimal or as all consuming as is appropriate for you at this time. However, all growth and change carries with it a certain amount of fear, as is often with the unknown. I encourage you to accept this as part of the process and proceed anyway. Also, the process of change or transformation can seem overwhelming at times, especially if you want or expect your transformative process to be substantial.

The process begins in the starting, and in the openness and willingness you bring to the starting. One of the most fundamental aspects of transformation through internal experience is that when you consciously work on changing your reactive and response patterns, your brain begins to process differently. When your brain begins to process differently, a whole host of positive changes result without conscious intent. Like the process of preparing the soil for a garden, if you put enough love, attention, and preparation into the soil and then plant a seed, a beautiful flower begins to blossom. You are not actually responsible for the creation of the flower. That happens on its own. However, creating the necessary conditions facilitates its growth. In this case, through intentional internal development, the process of transformation unfolds automatically. That is the miracle of turning inward. That is the miracle of cultivating higher internal experience. Have faith in the process and understand the science of transformation.

Along the path there will be questions and issues. Looking inward for guidance can be an invaluable tool. The following activity encourages a step-by-step process of change using the incredibly beneficial process of self-reflection through personal writing. This process is a powerful tool. It is designed to be used whenever you are faced with a challenge or issue and feel directed personal reflection would be beneficial.

Reflective Problem Solving
EXERCISE AND REFLECTION #19

Pick a problem, issue, or challenge in your life for which you would like to find a solution. Explain the problem or issue in as much detail as possible. In their book *Presence: An Explanation of Profound Change in People, Organizations, and Society,* Peter Senge, C. Otto Scharmer, Joseph Jaworski, and Betty Sue Flowers suggest that when you can begin to explain a problem or challenge in as much detail as possible, the answer begins to emerge.[1] Uniting this concept with the power of reflective writing give us a powerful tool for effective change.

_____

_____

_____

_____

_____

_____

_____

_____

_____

_____

_____

_____

_____

_____

Now list and describe in detail three possible solutions to the problem.

Solution #1

_____

_____

_____

_____

_____

_____

_____

_____

_____

_____

_____

_____

_____

_____

Solution #2

Solution #3

Process and reflect, again in detail, the pros and cons of each, and pick which solution would be both the most effective and the one most reflective of a higher emotional response.

_____

_____

_____

_____

_____

_____

_____

_____

_____

_____

_____

_____

_____

Reflect and process on specific and concrete ways you can carry out this solution.

_____

_____

_____

_____

_____

_____

_____

_____

_____

_____

_____

_____

_____

_____

_____

_____

The Process of Change

The process of change may not always go as expected, sometimes to the point that we begin to doubt its validity. The key is to focus on the internal, know that deep and fundamental change comes from routinely and sincerely engaging in the process, and be patient. I had, at times, doubted and felt it was all "bull." My wise friend reminded me that "bull" made great fertilizer for growth, and I really had no choice but to proceed.

Be patient with the process. Understand that every time you make a choice to notice, refocus, and choose a higher emotional state, you are creating deep and fundamental changes in your brain, body, and psyche. Understand that limbo is OK, meaning that sometimes there is a necessary waiting period for growth to happen, sort of like the ripening of fruit. Also understand that growth comes when we are most ready for it. When growth is too rapid or when we are unprepared, change is usually not sustainable. The best we can do when we feel stuck or feel the process isn't happening fast enough is to go within and better prepare ourselves for the process and outcome of transformation.

Keep in mind that there may be—most certainly will be, if you are practicing techniques of mental training—substantial growth beyond your conscious awareness. It is taking place at a deep and fundamental level. Understand that the difference between a happy day and a frustrating or challenging day may be a simple shift to a higher emotional state, and these days, repeatedly one after another, create our lived experience.

Remember that practice of all the concepts presented in this book promotes change and that change encourages more practice, which promotes more change. You have the capabilities within you to take the negative spirals described early in this book and reverse them to positive spirals. You have the power within you to make foundational changes in your physiology, which promote foundational changes in your life.

The process requires willingness at a very deep level. It requires allowance, or permission to actually be different, and it takes constant growth. A garden is always in a state of growth or transformation, and the same must be true for us. Some people talk about the idea of a "honeymoon period" in personal growth. I believe this concept is a myth.

The analogy of the honeymoon period is that, early on in our transformative process, we are so consumed by the positive changes of transformation we are in a constant state of elation. I believe that honeymoon period is a time of elation because at that time we are most in touch with the constant stimulus of growth. I believe this type of contact and elation is a choice, and we may choose, by concerted effort, to routinely re-create those circumstances. Intentionally re-creating these circumstances and stimuli for growth helps us to relive the honeymoon period over and over. I also believe, by the way, this is possible in relationships. But again, this process takes intention, willingness, and allowance to create a higher level of happiness. I believe the honeymoon period only ends in relationships, and in life, because we are only willing to let ourselves be so happy, and we perpetuate that on which we focus.

Scientific American recently featured an article on what distinguishes the "expert mind" from other minds. In other words, why do some people develop to become far and above what we determine to be the limits of human intellectual capabilities in specific areas?

Research shows that those who achieve extraordinary capabilities or development are those who keep challenging themselves just beyond their current level of development.[2]

I believe this is also true of personal transformation. I believe the myth of the honeymoon period exists because many of us, once we reach a certain level of development, become complacent and adopt practices that keep us at that level instead of continually reaching "just beyond." Maybe we do this because we become complacent, maybe because we only are willing to reach a certain level of happiness or transformation. I believe with attention, and constant vigilance on creating and maintaining even higher levels of emotional focus or internal development, the honeymoon period can be relived over and over again.

As my friend John at the coffee shop says, "Living a life of integrity comes from being internally integrated." The process and techniques presented in this book are designed to give you internal coherence or internal integration. Living from this state, and living consistently with this state, allows you to live from integrity. The final steps of our journey, and what we bring from the labyrinth back out into the world, is a life of integrity based on a life of higher internal experience.

How do we begin to live a life of integrity? By making choices, small and large, that coincides with the level of our higher internal development. Now we begin to take the necessary steps to have our life reflect who we have become, to honor our uniqueness, and to honor our higher consciousness. The following activity is loosely built on one developed by Lakein.[3] It is directed at determining our deepest values and encouraging us to see how our lives are, or could be better, at reflecting these values.

Identifying Core Values
EXERCISE AND REFLECTION #20

This is a three-part exercise. The first part asks you to write what you would like someone to be able to say about you after you have passed on from this life. Write and reflect what you would like someone to be able to say at a memorial service celebrating your life.

_____

_____

_____

_____

_____

_____

_____

_____

_____

_____

_____

Now, reflect on and write about what you would do if you had a year left to live. The purpose of this writing is to reflect on the things you would spend your time on if you know your time is finite. In other words, don't write about "getting your affairs in order." Write about how you would spend that time if you were not ill and resources were no object.

_____

_____

_____

_____

_____

_____

_____

_____

_____

_____

_____

_____

_____

_____

Finally, reflect on what you have done in the past day, week, or month to support those values. In addition, think about specific steps you can take to incorporate more of these values into your life, and spend more of your time pursuing them.

If you don't feel these questions have gotten to the core of what's really important to you, process and reflect on (1) what you would consider your deepest values, and (2) specifics and concrete steps, big or small, that you can take to more effectively incorporate these values into your daily life. Remember, repeated experience, even down to the level or our physiology, creates who we become. In what specific ways can you bring these deeply held values into your repeated internal experience?

_____

_____

_____

_____

_____

_____

_____

_____

_____

_____

_____

_____

_____

Putting It Together

Now, as you are all of the way out of the labyrinth, it is time to focus on creating external change based on a higher internal experience. Much of that external change will come automatically. As you have engaged in this process of transformation, you have created fundamental changes in your physiology, your brain, and your psyche that will begin to determine your outer experience. Remember, the moment you are truly willing to see yourself in the positive outcome of any situation, you have begun the physiological process of creating the necessary conditions for that outcome.

Based on the previous exercise, focus your attention on what you believe are your most deeply held values. Now, how do you begin to create the external circumstances conducive to living a life based on those values? What concrete steps do you need to take to create positive and foundational change? In *Man's Search for Meaning*, Victor Frankle, who wrote from a Nazi concentration camp, basically concludes that the deepest meaning any one person can create in his or her own life is to listen to what resonates within.[4] What resonates within you? What circumstances do you need to create in your external life to foster this resonance?

As we noted in Chapter One, the challenge of the labyrinth is not about navigating the path, as the path is circular and continuous in nature. The real challenge is to have the courage to begin the walk. Now, we continue that challenge with taking all we have learned and incorporating it into our lives to move from contemplation to action in the transformative process. In closing, I'd like to paraphrase a statement by Jerry Hicks and Esther Hicks. They use the term *ineffable* to illustrate the difficulty of describing the nonphysical in physical words.[5] I believe the same is true for higher levels of internal experience: The higher the level of the experience, the less words are sufficient. However, even though it is almost impossible to describe the depth of internal experience in words, we must try.

Exploring and processing what this experience means for you is the first step in being able to honestly cultivate it. At this point the words need to be yours. Moving from contemplation to action in cultivating higher internal experience now requires less of me and more of you. You have the knowledge. You have the tools. Are you willing to use them?

Putting It Together
EXERCISE AND REFLECTION #21

Victor Frankle states that the deepest meaning any one person can create in his or her own life is to listen to what resonates within. A major component of this book has been the processing and reflecting as done through the suggested personal writing. This activity asks you to focus on what resonates within you and to focus on taking action. How can you best internalize and put into action the concepts presented in this book? Take an in-depth look at the entire process presented within these covers, and pay special attention to that which resonates in you. Next, develop in-depth and specific action plans. Process and reflect in a way that is appropriate for you, and remember the success of the transformative process is directly dependent on the attention, intention, and action you give it.

_____

_____

_____

_____

_____

_____

_____

_____

_____

_____

REFERENCES

1. Senge, P., C. O. Scharmer, J. Jaworski, and B. S. Flowers, *Presence: An Exploration of Profound Change in People, Organizations, and Society* (New York: Doubleday, 2004).

2. Ross, P. E., "The Expert Mind," *Scientific American* 295:2 (2006): 64–71.

3. Lakein, A., *How to Get Control of Your Time and Your Life* (New York: Signet, 1974).

4. Frankle, V., *Man's Search for Meaning* (Boston: Beacon, 1992).

5. Hicks, E., and J. Hicks, *Ask and It Is Given: Learning to Manifest Your Desires* (Carlsbad, CA: Hay House, 2004).

Alane Daugherty's passion, professional training, research, and teaching experience are grounded in health promotion, stress management, the psychophysiology of internal experience, and the neuroscience of transformation. She has received recognition for both her scientific research and her university teaching, and has taught courses at The Claremont Graduate University, Colorado College, The University of La Verne and California State Polytechnic University, Pomona. Dr. Daugherty routinely presents workshops and conducts seminars on these subjects at corporations, non-profit, and service learning organizations and has presented at a number of professional conferences including the American Educational Research Association, The Lilly conference on college and university teaching, and the American College of Sports Medicine. She is a member of the Golden Key national honor society, and is listed in the Manchester Who's Who honor's edition of executive and professional women. She received her Master's degree from Cal Poly Pomona with an emphasis in exercise science and her PhD from Claremont Graduate University. The title of her dissertation was "The physiological, cognitive and psycho-social effects of emotional refocusing: a summative and formative analysis."

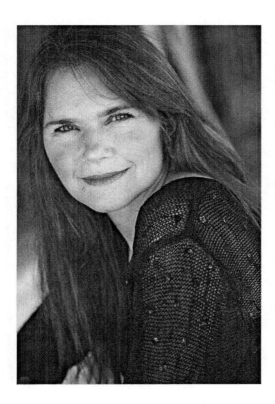